Vegan

Pregnancy Guide for First Time Mums

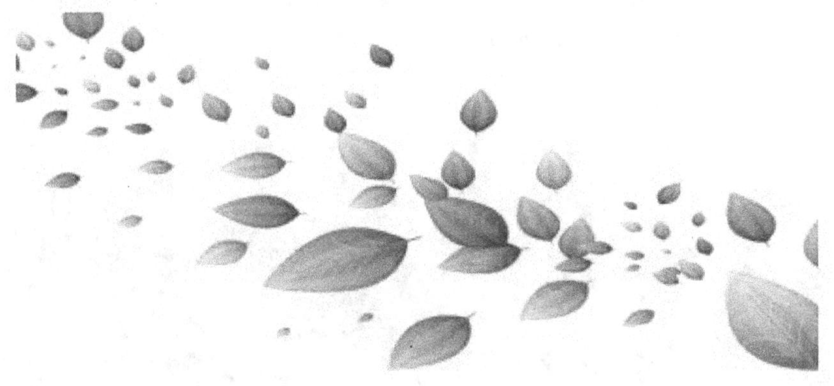

A Complete Nutritional Meal Plan for A Healthy Pregnancy.

Jennifer Osborne

Copyright © 2023 by Jennifer Osborne

All rights reserved.

This book is written as a source of information only. The information contained in this book is provided in good faith and is believed to be accurate and reliable as of the date of publication. The author does not assume any responsibility for any errors or omissions that may appear.

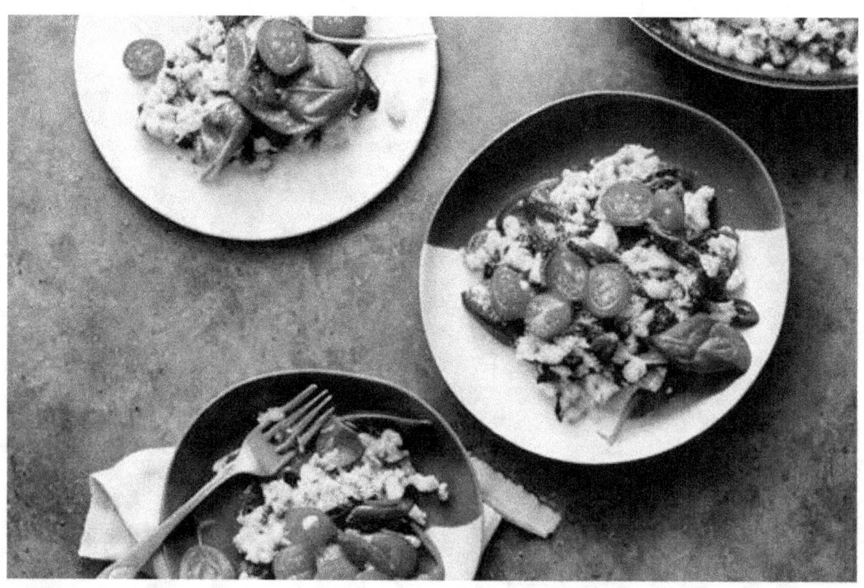

Table of Content

About The Book

Congratulations, you're expecting a Baby!! Whether you're vegan or just looking to make sure your pregnancy diet is as healthy as possible, Vegan Pregnancy for Mum is here to help. With 40+ delicious recipes and easy-to-follow nutritional guidelines, this cookbook will make sure you and your baby get all the essential nutrients to stay strong and healthy during this special time. Get ready for a happy, healthy pregnancy with Vegan Pregnancy for Mum!

Want to ensure your baby gets the best nutrition while in the womb? As a first-time mom, you want to make sure you're doing everything right for your baby's health. Eating the right foods during pregnancy is essential for your baby's development, but it can be difficult to know what to eat and how much. Everything First-Time Moms Need to Know About Eating While Pregnant provides a comprehensive guide that simplifies the process and helps you make the best choices for both you and your baby.

This guide is designed to make eating during pregnancy easier and more enjoyable by providing easy-to-understand information about nutrition, meal planning, food safety, and more. With this guide, you can rest assured that you are doing everything possible to give your little one the best start in life! Start making informed decisions today! Learn everything first-time moms need to know about eating while pregnant.

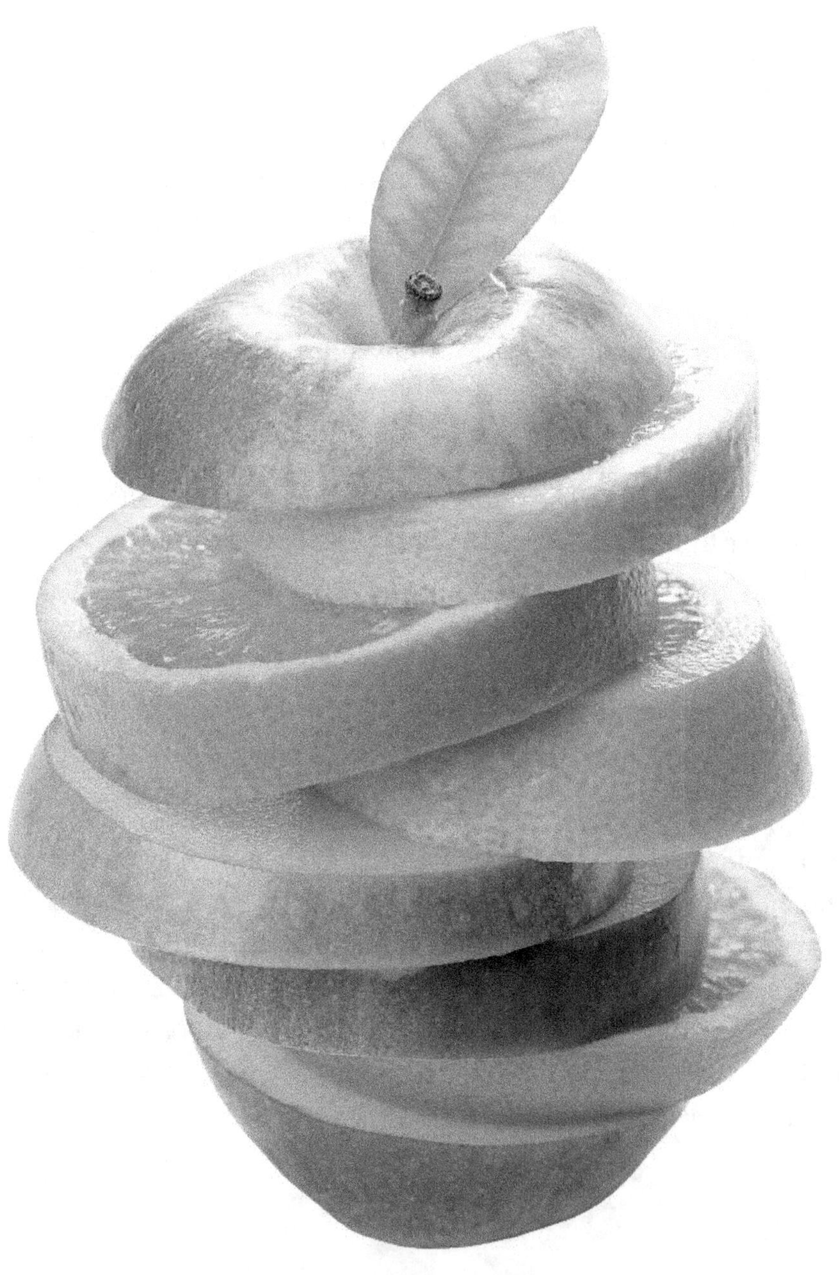

Introduction

Vegan Pregnancy Guide for First-Time Mums

Congratulations on finding out you're pregnant! After the initial shock and joy wear off, you may be considering what you can do to help support this new life. Doctors may have advised you to avoid certain foods, abstain from alcohol, and consume less caffeine, but I doubt anyone has yet to advise you on the best things to consume. Did you know that healthy nutrition during pregnancy can boost your baby's IQ, lower the likelihood that they will become ill or obese in the future, make labor less difficult and painful, and hasten your recovery after giving birth? The goal of pregnancy and labor preparation is frequently to reduce risks. Continue reading to find out how to give your child the best start in life.

Why Is Eating Well While Pregnant Important?

An ideal diet is crucial for a healthy pregnancy, to avoid problems, and even after delivery. A nutritious diet during pregnancy has been found to lower your baby's risk of developing obesity, diabetes, and heart disease later in life.

Additionally, eating healthfully and using specific probiotics throughout your pregnancy can significantly lower the likelihood that your unborn child will have asthma, eczema, or hay fever (more on this later).

This month-by-month pregnancy diet guide and chart lists important foods to concentrate on each month for the growth of the unborn child, as well as typical physical symptoms encountered during this period and dietary and lifestyle tips to manage them.

Let's first take a look at some basic recommendations for a healthy diet during your entire pregnancy before diving into each month.

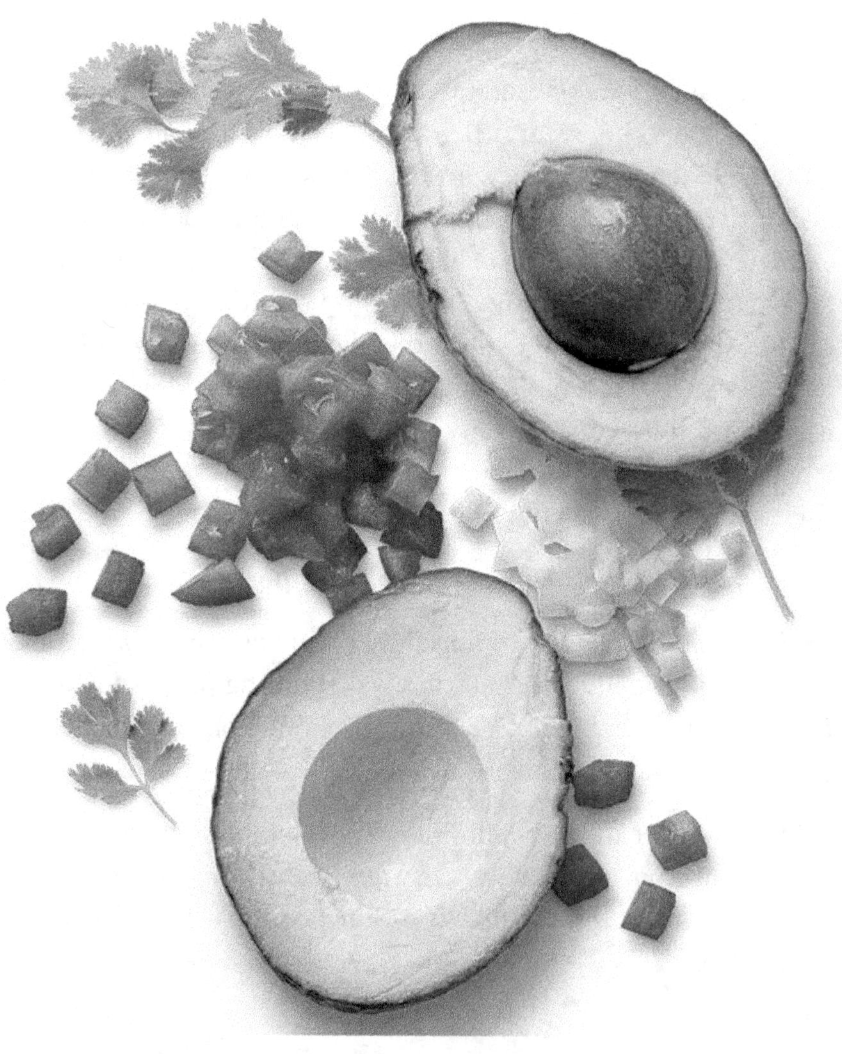

Chapter One

Recommendations For Eating During the Whole Pregnancy

Focus on whole foods that are high in nutrients; these should be as raw and unprocessed as possible. When buying packaged foods, a good rule of thumb is to stay away from anything with ingredients you are unsure of. The majority of expectant women require 80 grams (2.8 oz) of high-quality protein daily. The best sources of protein are those that have undergone less processing and are, if at all feasible, grass-fed, free-range, or organic. Calculate the recommended daily intake of protein in grams by multiplying your pre-pregnancy weight by 1.2. (For example, a 65 kg woman requires 78g of protein per day.)

Adequate healthy fats: In contrast to much of the now outdated government advice to reduce fats, modern research is confirming the importance of healthy fats for all body systems. Proper fat consumption throughout pregnancy is crucial for the unborn child's organ and brain development. If you choose to eat them, olive oil, avocados, nuts and seeds, eggs, oily seafood, and meats are all excellent sources of fat.

A lot of fresh, nutritious fruits and vegetables that are high in fiber, vitamins, and minerals. Eating a variety of fruits and vegetables will provide your body with the majority of the nutrients it needs, as well as a lot of fiber to keep you from getting constipated. Focus on consuming a lot of leafy green vegetables (parsley, kale, spinach, collard greens) for a high-quality source of folate, like ten or more glasses of beverages each day. It's critical to drink enough water throughout pregnancy to replenish the baby's amniotic fluid, prevent morning sickness, and prevent constipation due to the rapid increase in blood volume. Ideal sources of most of this fluid should be juices, herbal tea, and water. Steer clear of alcohol, soft drinks, as well as excessive amounts of tea and coffee.

Avoid processed, packaged, and high-sugar foods as they often include chemicals that are harmful to both you and your unborn child and offer very little in the way of nutrition. You won't feel deprived if you replace low-nutrient foods with healthy, satiating whole foods.

Moderate amounts of grains and starches: Choose whole grains like brown rice, whole oats, quinoa, or whole-grain pasta when consuming grains. Beetroot, sweet potato, pumpkin, and parsnip all have nutrient-dense carbohydrates. Aim for moderate servings of carbohydrates at each meal because excessive ingestion of carbohydrates (especially refined carbs and sugars) during pregnancy might disrupt blood sugar levels and lead to gestational diabetes.

Supplements To Think About While Pregnant

This is only a general recommendation; before starting any of the indicated supplements, see your doctor.

A high-quality prenatal multivitamin that has at least 400 mcg of Throughout the whole nine months of pregnancy, but especially during the first four weeks while the spinal cord is developing, it is critical to take a high-quality prenatal multivitamin that contains at least 400 mcg of folic acid (to help prevent neural tube defects). As soon as you realize you are pregnant, or ideally before you start trying to conceive, you must get started.

You may benefit more from taking supplements of folinic acid and/or 5-MTHF if you are aware of an MTHFR gene mutation, which regulates how folic acid is converted into other substances needed by the body.

Lactobacillus Rhamnosus, a probiotic. Between 60 and 80% of babies with both parents having a history of eczema are likely to develop it. It has been demonstrated that taking Lactobacillus rhamnosus throughout the last trimester of pregnancy (and occasionally postnatally) significantly lowers the risk of the unborn child developing atopy (asthma, eczema, hay fever). Consult your doctor about if this probiotic may be beneficial for you if you or your partner have a history of allergies.

The development of a fetus's bones and teeth depends on magnesium, which can also stop the uterus from contracting too early. Additionally, it's a fantastic vitamin to take throughout pregnancy because it eases muscle tension, which can help with constipation, support tissue growth, and encourage sound sleep.

The development of your baby's neurological and visual systems as well as the production of breast milk depends on fish oil and omega-3 fatty acids. Studies have indicated that taking omega-3 supplements while pregnant can improve your baby's cognitive development and raise their IQ in the future. A larger consumption of omega-3 fatty acids may reduce the likelihood of an infant developing allergies, according to other studies. Omega-3 fatty acids have also been proven to minimize the incidence of preeclampsia, early labor, and maternal depression. Talk to your doctor if you believe an omega-3 supplement will be beneficial for you, but bear in mind that the quality of these supplements varies substantially. Instead of choosing the cheapest brand on the shelves of your neighborhood pharmacy, choose those with a reputation for purity and proper storage.

Month 1 of the Pregnant Diet

The Growth of a Baby:

Your baby is an embryo made up of two layers of cells throughout the first month of pregnancy. From here, all the body's organs and parts will develop. The neural tube develops during this month, which is why it's so important to take folic acid supplements (or folinic acid, or 5-MTHF, if you know you have an MTHFR gene mutation) to avoid neural tube problems.

Personal Symptoms:

Early on in pregnancy, morning sickness is frequently experienced. Not all women experience it, but for some, it can be very severe. The good news is that by the start of their second trimester, most women report that their morning sickness has subsided.

Here are several methods to lessen nausea, which can strike at any time of day and not just in the morning:

- 15 to 20 minutes before getting out of bed in the morning, eat a snack high in carbohydrates to help settle your stomach before you start to move around.

- Try keeping some plain bread or crackers beside your bed so you may have them when you wake up.

- Eat smaller, more frequent meals (i.e., 6 meals a day, rather than 3). Avoid being overly hungry in between meals.

- Pick simple-to-digest meals for your diet.

- Try to drink more liquids than food in between meals.

- Avoid eating fried, high-fat, and spicy foods because they can make you feel sicker.

- When you feel queasy, sip ordinary soda water throughout the day.

Key Foods to Pay Attention to in the First Month of Pregnancy:

Green leafy vegetables like spinach, rocket, and parsley, nutritious grains, and legumes are foods high in folate (lentils, beans, chickpeas)

Early pregnancy morning sickness and vomiting can be effectively treated naturally with vitamin B6: 40 mg given twice a day. If you think taking this supplement would be beneficial, discuss it with your doctor.

- Avoid eating raw or undercooked meats when pregnant.
- Cold cured meat slices
- Sashimi or sushi is raw seafood.
- Supple cheeses
- Sushi bars
- An uncooked egg (and foods that contain them e.g., Mayonnaise and raw cake batter)
- Raw fruits and vegetables
- High caffeine content (coffee, black tea)

Month 2 of the Pregnant Diet

The Growth of a Baby:

Your baby has distinct, slightly webbed fingers and is about the size of a kidney bean in the second month of pregnancy.

Personal Symptoms:

In the second month, nausea and exhaustion are frequent.

Key Vegetables to Eat in The Second Month of Pregnancy:

Ginger for nausea: Studies have shown that ginger relieves nausea just as effectively as the most popular anti-nausea medications. Try shredding two tablespoons of ginger into boiling water for tea, munching on crystallized ginger candies all day, or cooking with ginger powder.

Low vitamin E status was linked in this study to an increased risk of miscarriage.

These are some good sources of vitamin E:

- Fresh almonds
- Avocado
- Olive juice
- Sunburst seeds
- Hazelnuts

Month 3 Pregnancy Diet

The Growth of a Baby:

Your baby is roughly 7 to 8 cm (3 inches) long and weighs the same as a pea pod in the third month of pregnancy. Now, tiny, individual fingerprints can be recognized.

Personal Symptoms:

Normally, the nausea subsides by the end of this month. Read this endearing article about one woman's struggle with crippling morning sickness and the lessons she discovered along the way to help you get through.

Key Foods to Pay Attention to In the Third Month of Pregnancy:

To keep you and your baby hydrated, be sure to consume at least 10 glasses of water every day in addition to fluid-rich fruits and vegetables.

Month 4 Diet for Pregnancy

The Growth of a Baby:

Greetings from the second trimester! Your baby weighs 140g and measures about 13 cm (5.5 inches) long in the fourth month of pregnancy (5oz). The skeleton is transitioning from squishy cartilage to bone through hardening. This month is usually when your baby bump starts to appear.

Physical Symptoms:

This month, you may notice that you have more energy and that your nausea has subsided.

Key Foods to Include in Your Diet During the Fourth Month of Pregnancy:

Iron-rich foods: Your blood volume will have increased by 50% by the time you give birth. Increase your consumption of high-quality proteins, such as eggs and free-range meats (organic or grass-fed whenever possible). Vegetarians should consume iron-rich plant foods such as leafy greens and legumes with each meal, along with a source of vitamin C (such as a squeeze of lemon juice or some capsicum/peppers), as this improves the body's absorption of iron from non-animal sources.

If you've been feeling extremely tired or suspect there's a problem with your iron intake, talk to your doctor about taking supplements. Pregnancy iron deficiency can lead to low birth weight, iron-deficient newborns, and fatigue for the mother.

The Pregnancy Diet Week 5

The Development of a Baby:

In the fifth month of pregnancy, you'll be able to see your baby's elbows and eyelids. The baby is approximately 10.5 inches (27 cm) long. You usually have more energy this month, and it's pretty obvious that you're pregnant by now. You might start to feel the baby move around this month!

Physical Symptoms;

Bloating and fluid retention may be an issue this month. Avoid excessive salt and processed foods, and make sure to drink plenty of water.

Key Foods to Include in Your Diet During The Fifth Month:

During pregnancy, calcium is essential for your developing baby's teeth and bones, as well as the development of a healthy heart, nervous system, and muscles.

Several excellent calcium sources (at least two per day) include:

- Sardines are small fish with bones.
- Almonds

- Tahini
- Green leafy vegetables
- (If tolerated) dairy

Because your body cannot store vitamin C, it is critical to consume it daily through foods such as broccoli, tomatoes, and oranges. Throughout pregnancy, vitamin C is required for the production of collagen, a protein that provides structure to cartilage, tendons, bones, and skin as well as aiding your body in the fight against infections.

Month Six Pregnancy Diet

The Development of a Baby:

The average baby weight in the sixth month of pregnancy is 660g (1.5 lb). As the baby grows in weight, his or her wrinkly skin begins to sag.

Physical Symptoms:

Hunger is more common this month. While extra calories are required to support your baby's rapid growth, choose foods that are high in nutrients rather than calories to provide you and your baby with the nutrients required for healthy growth.

Constipation is common during this time. Constipation is a common pregnancy symptom because the body slows digestion to ensure optimal nutrient uptake to aid in the growth of your baby. Because the body's nutritional requirements are met, focusing on a whole-food, nutrient-dense diet is likely to prevent constipation. If you suffer from constipation, focus on eating a lot of whole grains, fiber-rich fruits, vegetables, and legumes, as well as drinking plenty of water throughout the day.

Key Vegetables to Eat In The Sixth Month of Pregnancy:

Eat more whole grains, fruits, vegetables, and legumes to avoid constipation. Aim for 25-30g of fiber per day. This amounts to about 2 cups of wheat bran, 2 cups of beans, or 5 large apples. Use this tool to calculate your daily fiber intake from common foods.

As a natural remedy for constipation, take 1 tablespoon of psyllium dissolved in a glass of water before bed to encourage a good bowel movement the next morning.

The Seventh Week of The Pregnancy Diet

The Development of a Baby:

Hello from the third trimester! During the seventh month of pregnancy, your baby has grown to a length of more than 40 cm (15 inches). They can open and close their eyes and observe their surroundings.

Personal Symptoms:

Heartburn: As your uterus expands, pressure on the stomach increases, causing acid to rise into the esophagus.

Here are some tips for avoiding heartburn:

- Regularly eat modest meals.
- Avoid fried, high-fat, and spicy foods.
- Consume no more than 80% of your calories.
- After eating, avoid lying down for 45 minutes.
- To avoid going to bed straight after dinner, try to have dinner earlier.
- Consider raising the head of your bed at night.

These Are the Key Vegetables to Eat in The Seventh Month of Pregnancy:

Protein: Getting enough protein throughout pregnancy is critical to the development of the fetus. Most women require 80 grams of protein (2.8 oz) per day for a healthy pregnancy. This amount of protein should be consumed daily to lower your risk of preeclampsia, morning sickness, and other complications. It's critical to get enough high-quality protein because low-protein diets can increase the baby's risk of developing high blood pressure. Use this protein calorie meter to ensure you get enough protein each day.

Month 8 Pregnancy Diet

The Development of a Baby:

The baby weighs approximately 2.4 kg at the moment (4.7lb). Lungs have fully formed, and fat layers are expanding.

Physical Symptoms:

You may experience frequent urination, backaches, shortness of breath, and difficulty sleeping as your pregnancy progresses. Consider taking a warm shower before bed and purchasing a long pillow to support your stomach as you sleep on your side.

Key Foods to Include in Your Diet During the Eighth Month of Pregnancy:

The omega-3 fatty acids: Because the third trimester is when a baby's brain grows and develops the fastest, include omega-3 sources in your diet, such as:

- Fatty fish like salmon

- Nuts and seeds
- Flaxseed pulverized

Sour cherries have been shown to promote sound sleep by increasing your body's natural production of melatonin (our sleep-regulating hormone). Try drinking 1 cup of unsweetened cherry juice before bed to improve your sleep.

Pregnancy Diet for Month 9

The Development of a Baby:

The baby is almost ready to come out. At delivery, they typically weigh around 3.4kg and measure more than 51cm (20.5 inches) from head to toe (7.5lb).

Personal Significance:

Swollen hands and feet are common in the last month. To avoid excessive salt consumption, drink plenty of water. Try a light activity like swimming or walking to promote fluid mobility.

Key Vegetables to Eat in The Ninth Month of Genesis:

Garlic: A "heavy" garlic intake during the final month of pregnancy has been linked to a significantly lower incidence of premature labor. This is thought to be related to garlic's antibacterial properties, which help to reduce infections of the vaginal and urinary systems, which can lead to preterm birth. What is the best option? A "high" garlic intake was defined in this study as consuming 1 clove per week.

Dates: Eating six dates every day for the last four weeks before the expected due date increased the likelihood of spontaneous labor (i.e., reduced the need for an inducement), encouraged greater cervical dilation, accelerated the first stage of labor, and reduced the need for medical and pharmaceutical intervention. According to a second, more recent study that supported the first's findings, date consumption in late pregnancy is a safe supplement to consider because it reduces the need for labor intervention without having any negative effects on the mother or child.

Dates are a tasty natural sweetener that can be used in recipes or as a snack throughout the day.

Raisins: Consuming two handfuls of dried raisins per week has been linked to a lower risk of preterm labor, similar to garlic. Try munching on raisins to add a sweet flavor boost to salads or rice dishes.

Eating well during pregnancy can have a significant and long-term impact on your pregnancy and delivery experience, as well as your baby's health and development. I was inspired to write this guide because there is so little reliable information available about eating healthfully while pregnant. Based on the facts, it will assist you in providing your child with the best possible start in life.

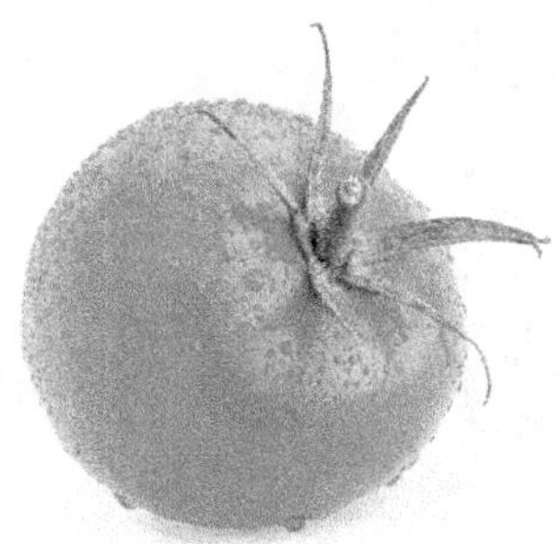

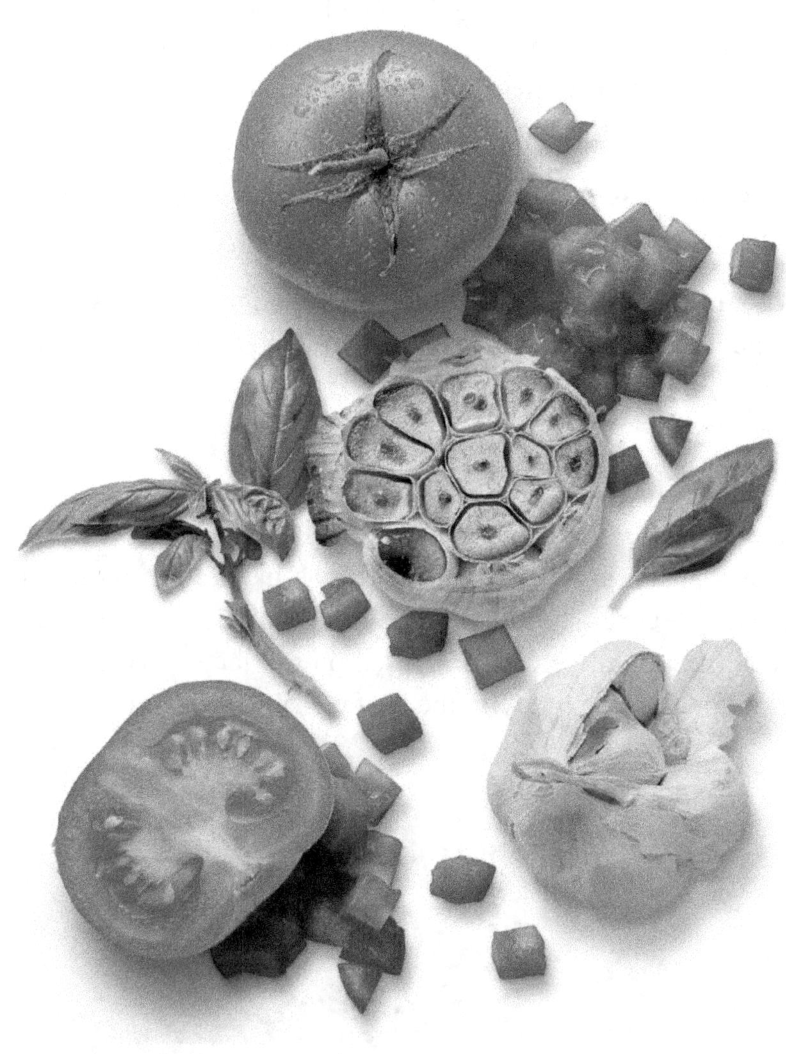

Chapter Two

What To Know About Food Cravings During Pregnancy

Pregnancy is one of the most significant physical changes you will ever experience. And, yes, practically every aspect of your body undergoes some sort of change. However, you will notice that your appetite changes, often significantly, before all of this occurs—possibly even before you receive a positive pregnancy test.

Certain foods that you used to enjoy will become unbearably unpleasant when you are pregnant. There may also be foods that you yearn for that you have never tried before. You may find yourself suddenly craving strange combinations of goods. Pickles and ice cream are probably the most well-known pregnancy pairing, but they are only the tip of the iceberg.

Let's look more closely at pregnancy cravings, including their causes, frequency, typical foods that pregnant people seem to crave, and when and whether they are cause for concern.

Pregnancy Food Cravings: Myth or Reality?

Although experts are unsure why pregnancy makes you crave certain foods (and despise others), they are certain that it does. According to one study, 50% to 90% of pregnant women in the

United States experience food cravings at some point during their pregnancy.

When Do Pregnancy Cravings Begin?

Although every pregnant woman is different, pregnancy cravings typically begin near the end of the first trimester, peak in the second trimester, and then begin to fade as the third trimester concludes.

However, because breastfeeding and pregnancy both require more calories, breastfeeding parents may develop cravings of their own and will undoubtedly continue to have larger appetites.

Why Do Food Cravings Occur During Pregnancy?

There are a few basic hypotheses as to why pregnancy alters our taste buds and causes us to prefer certain foods. Here are some of the most popular theories

Hormonal Changes

During pregnancy, there are significant hormonal changes, especially in the first trimester. Consider PMS multiplied by a million. Pregnancy hormones may alter the types of desires you have, similar to what happens when you anticipate your period. Hormones can affect your sensory perception of food, sense of smell, and mood, which will change the types of meals you crave.

Sensational Shifts

Many expectant mothers claim that during pregnancy, they develop bloodhound-like senses, able to detect odors from a distance but easily overwhelmed by them. As a result, our cravings for certain foods may change. Foods with overpowering aromas may turn people off completely. Foods with pleasant, fragrant aromas may also pique people's interest.

Nutritional Requirements are Changing

Pregnant women require more nutrients such as calcium and iron. As a result, you may begin to crave foods containing these components. The only problem is that your body may misinterpret your calcium requirement as a desire for an enormous container of vanilla ice cream. Eat the ice cream. However, remember to include more nutrient-dense sources of the vitamin you're looking for in your diet. In terms of calcium, dark leafy greens, almonds, and seafood are all excellent sources, in addition to that well-deserved ice cream.

Surviving on the Strongest

Some of our desires and dislikes are motivated by a desire to protect ourselves and our growing children. Many of us, for example, discover that items like coffee and alcohol that are unhealthy or less healthy naturally make their way to our lists of aversions. The argument is that eating meat increases the risk of bacterial contamination, which causes many of us to lose interest in it. However, these are not the experiences of all pregnant women.

A Yearning for Coziness

Many of us simply crave comfort foods, such as sweets and carbohydrates. We may also long for childhood favorites that bring us joy and love. When we are experiencing morning sickness during pregnancy, we may yearn for the foods we frequently eat.

Preferences Regarding Culture

One of the most intriguing aspects of cravings is how our individual preferences for specific meals can be influenced by our upbringing. When it comes to PMS, American women seem to crave chocolate the most, whereas Japanese women crave rice. The same tendencies apply when it comes to cravings during pregnancy.

Most Popular Food Cravings During Pregnancy

When it comes to cravings during pregnancy, there is a wide range of variations. Some people have extremely unusual desires that appear out of nowhere. However, experts have identified certain trends in American women's cravings during pregnancy. According to one study, the following are the most common pregnancy cravings:

Sweets, flavorful carbs with a lot of calories, such as pizza or chips, and meat-based proteins, Fruits.

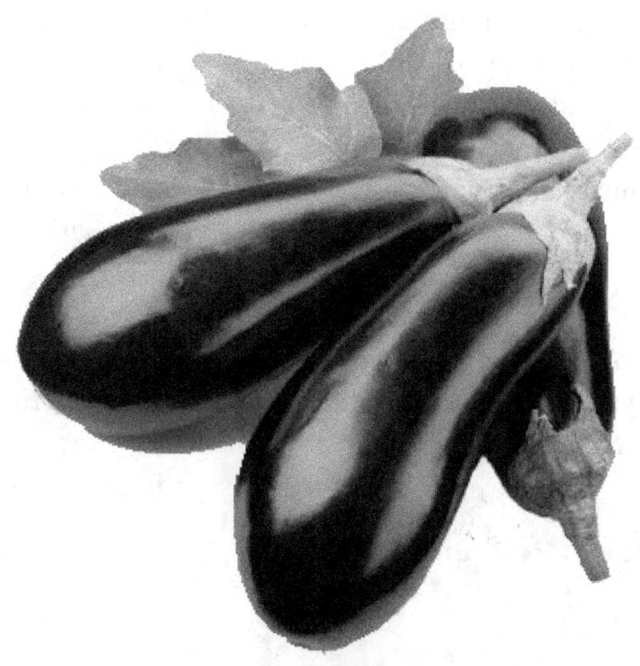

Chapter Three

How To Maintain a Healthy Relationship with Food While Pregnant.

In general, there is no reason not to indulge your pregnancy cravings as long as less nutritious items are consumed in moderation and your diet is varied and nutrient-rich overall. Dieting during pregnancy is never a good idea, but it is also a good time to focus as much as possible on making healthy choices. A healthy, balanced diet will keep you and your child healthy and ensure that you are ready for labor and the postpartum period. You will need more calories during pregnancy. While pregnant, you will need 500 more calories per day on average, but this can vary. Rather than focusing on the quantity, try to pay attention to your hunger cues.

You'll need more of a few nutrients to help your baby grow and keep your body healthy.

Calcium

You should consume 1,000 milligrams of calcium per day while pregnant. Calcium is found in dairy products, dark leafy greens, fish, fortified cereals and drinks, nuts, and sesame seeds.

B6 vitamin

Folic acid is required for both your increased blood supply during pregnancy and your baby's protection against neural tube abnormalities. Citrus fruits, almonds, green leafy vegetables, beans, and lentils, as well as prenatal vitamins, contain folic acid.

Iron

You will need more iron during pregnancy, with a daily requirement of around 27 milligrams. If you develop anemia while pregnant, you must consume iron-rich foods like whole grains, meats, dark leafy greens, beans, and nuts, as well as a supplement. Nonheme iron, which is found in plant-based foods, is more difficult to absorb than heme iron, which is found in animal foods. As a result, you should exercise extreme caution when obtaining iron. If you drink tea or coffee with your meals, your body may have a harder time absorbing iron from the vegetables. Instead, combine an iron-rich diet with a vitamin C-rich food, such as orange juice, tomato sauce, or broccoli, to help your body better absorb this mineral.

A blood test will be performed early in your pregnancy to determine your iron level. If your iron levels are low, your doctor may advise you to take an iron supplement. Anemia caused by a lack of iron can be dangerous for both you and your unborn child (like preterm birth). If you suspect you may be suffering from anemia symptoms such as fatigue, weakness, pale or yellow skin, cold hands and feet, dizziness, or lightheadedness, consult your doctor immediately.

Protein

During pregnancy, you'll need more protein than usual—75 grams on average per day. Protein can be found in a variety of foods, including meats, fish, eggs, almonds, peas, beans, and soy products.

Protein is essential for your growing child's development because it (Servings:) as the foundation for cells. It is made up of amino acids, nine of which are essential and cannot be produced by your body on its own. Animal foods contain roughly twice as much protein per serving (approximately 20 grams) as plant foods (10 grams or less). Furthermore, unlike animal foods, plant foods do not contain all nine essential amino acids. Because of this, it is critical to obtain protein from a variety of vegetarian sources, preferably including a protein-rich item in each meal.

In the second and third trimesters, you'll need 70 grams per day. (Note: Your protein requirements may vary depending on your weight, level of activity, and medical history)

Vegetarian protein sources that are suitable include:

- Eggs, dairy products, Lentils, kidney beans, and chickpeas are examples of legumes.
- Soy products include tofu, tempeh, soy milk, and soybeans.
- There are numerous nut butter, seeds, and nuts (such as peanuts, almonds, cashews, chia seeds, flaxseed, and walnuts)

Zinc

You'll need 11 milligrams per day. Because your body has no way of storing zinc, you'll need a consistent dose to help with growth during pregnancy. Because plant foods are less effective at absorbing zinc, animal foods are the best sources of zinc. As a result, vegans and vegetarians have a more difficult time getting enough zinc from food alone. Consume a variety of zinc-rich plant foods and ensure that your prenatal supplement contains zinc.

You can meet your zinc requirements by eating a variety of iron-rich foods. Foods high in zinc include:

- Fortified breakfast cereals
- Beans
- Whey protein, soy products, whole grains, seeds, and nuts
- Yogurt with oats, milk, and cheese

Calcium

You will need 1,000 mg per day. Calcium both strengthens and protects your infant's bones. In reality, your bones will be used to supplement what your child does not get from the foods you eat, particularly during the last trimester, which increases your risk of osteoporosis.

One serving of most dairy products and fortified soy milk provides about one-third of your daily calcium requirements. The calcium content of the remaining plant-based and fortified foods on the list below is 100 mg or less per serving. If you're not sure if a product contains calcium, look at the label. You may be able to get all of the calcium you need from your diet if you consume dairy products. If your prenatal vitamin does not contain calcium (some do not, and many only contain 100 to 200 grams), talk to your provider about taking a calcium supplement.

Try to eat multiple portions of the calcium-rich foods listed below every day:

- Milk, yogurt, and cheese
- Breakfast cereals, orange juice, and calcium-fortified almond or soy milk
- chickpeas, lentils, and white beans
- Almonds, tahini, and sesame seeds
- Figs in tins
- Tofu cathodic (look for calcium chloride or calcium sulfate on the ingredients list)
- Some green vegetables, such as kale, turnip greens, mustard greens, broccoli, and bok choy, are high in calcium (others, such as spinach and beet greens, contain calcium, but your body does not absorb it as well).

Vitamin D

You must get 600 IU or more of vitamin D every day.

This vitamin helps your body absorb calcium, which helps your baby's bones grow. When you are exposed to the sun, even for a short time, your body produces vitamin D. The best source of vitamin D is fatty fish, but it can also be found in a few vegetarian meals, including:

- Egg whites
- Fortified cow's milk cereals
- Plant kinds of milk
- Vitamin-fortified orange juice.

Even so, supplements may be necessary, especially in the winter. Several prenatal supplements contain vitamin D as well. If yours does not, you should talk to your doctor about taking a vitamin D supplement.

Vitamin B12

You'll need 2.6 mcg per day. Your baby's brain development is heavily reliant on vitamin B12, which is only found naturally in animal diets. If you consume multiple servings of dairy foods per day, you should get enough calcium.

If you are vegan and avoid dairy, you must consume vitamin B12-fortified foods (be sure to check for fortification on the product label).

Vitamin B12-containing foods include:

Other plant milks, such as breakfast cereals made from soy

If you don't consume fortified dairy products or meals regularly and your prenatal supplement doesn't contain B12, your doctor will probably advise you to take a separate vitamin B12 supplement.

Iodine

Every day, you must take 220 mcg. Iodine is necessary for the development of your baby's brain and central nervous system, as well as for the production of specific hormones by your thyroid. Low iodine levels may result in hypothyroidism or goiter (an enlarged thyroid)

DHA

A daily dose of 200 mg DHA is required. When you are pregnant, DHA is an omega-3 fatty acid that helps your unborn child's eyes and brain grow. According to some research, it may also help to reduce the risk of premature birth. It can be found in fish, fish oil, and microalgae.

Although the body can convert ALA, another type of omega-3 fatty acid found in chia and flax seeds, into DHA, the process is ineffective. DHA is added to a variety of juices, soy beverages, and yogurt. Taking an omega-3 supplement made from algae, on the other hand, is by far the simplest way for vegetarians and vegans to get the recommended amount of DHA.

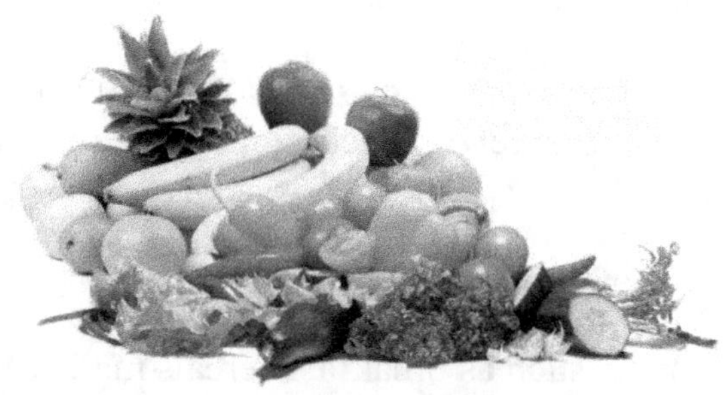

Chapter Four

Meal Plan and Vegetarian Pregnancy Diets

Is it safe to become pregnant while vegetarian or vegan?

You can have a safe pregnancy whether you're a vegetarian or vegan if you prepare properly. You can get all the nutrition you need without eating meat, fish, or chicken (or animal products like eggs and dairy if you're vegan), as long as you eat a variety of nutritious vegetarian meals that include important nutrients for your baby's cellular, brain, and organ development.

In reality, a well-planned plant-based diet is rich in nutrients such as fiber, vitamins, and minerals, all of which promote both your baby's development and your health. Furthermore, it contains little saturated fat and cholesterol, both of which are harmful in excess even if you are not pregnant. Inform your healthcare practitioner about your nutrition during your first prenatal or preconception visit. If you follow a vegan diet, you may want to consult with a dietician.

To ensure you get enough of what you need, you may need to supplement your prenatal vitamin with fortified foods and take certain supplements on occasion. Prior to ingesting any supplements while pregnant, always check with your doctor.

Pregnancy diets that are vegetarian or vegan

You can satisfy your nutritional requirements while pregnant as a vegetarian or vegan by consistently including the following foods in your meals: nuts, seeds, legumes, soy products, and fortified foods (along with dairy and eggs if you eat them).

Can I remain a vegetarian or vegan while nursing?

It is unquestionably possible to nurse while following a vegetarian or vegan diet. Many of the same nutritional guidelines from pregnancy apply when nursing to help your body meet the demands of milk production.

Again, the nutrients to concentrate on are:

- Protein consumption of 70 grams per day
- Calcium intake of 1,000 mg per day
- 2.8 mcg of B12 per day and 10 mg of iron per day
- 13 milligrams of zinc per day
- Every day, take 600 IU of vitamin D.
- DHA 200 mg/day
- 290 micrograms of iodine per day

To get many of these nutrients, keep taking your prenatal vitamins and eating the same foods you did during pregnancy. It is critical to maintain a healthy diet throughout your pregnancy because it will benefit both you and your unborn child. Eating a well-balanced diet is essential for your baby's development as well as your overall health.

Although being pregnant is an extremely joyful experience, it can also be extremely taxing, so it's critical to provide your body with the nutrients it requires to perform at its best. Many pregnant women wonder what they should and should not eat. The recommendations for a healthy diet during pregnancy are generally the same as they were before you became pregnant. It is critical to become acquainted with the foods that must be consumed in moderation while pregnant. Furthermore, it is critical to maintain strict food cleanliness standards and ensure that the food you eat has been thoroughly cooked.

While pregnant, a diverse, balanced diet should include a variety of foods such as:

- A variety of vitamin-rich fruits and vegetables
- Starchy foods such as potatoes, whole-grain bread, and noodles
- Eggs, salmon, and pulses are examples of protein-rich lean foods.
- Dairy products high in calcium

If you're stuck for dinner ideas and need some mealtime inspiration, this book can help. Continue reading to discover 24 delectable, nutritious dishes high in vitamins and minerals. Using these meal suggestions, you can easily transition from breakfast to dinner.

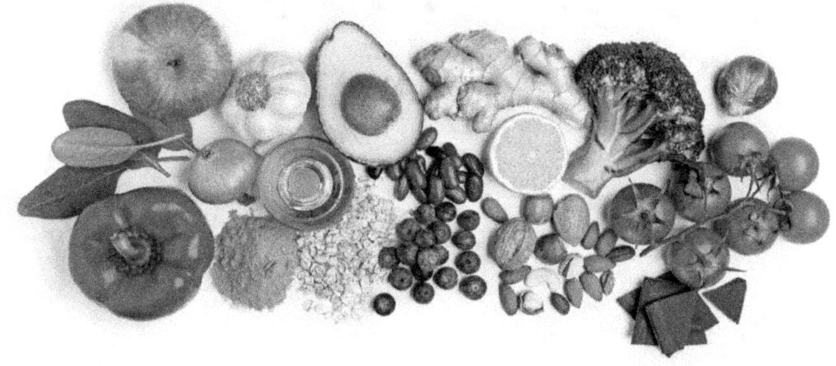

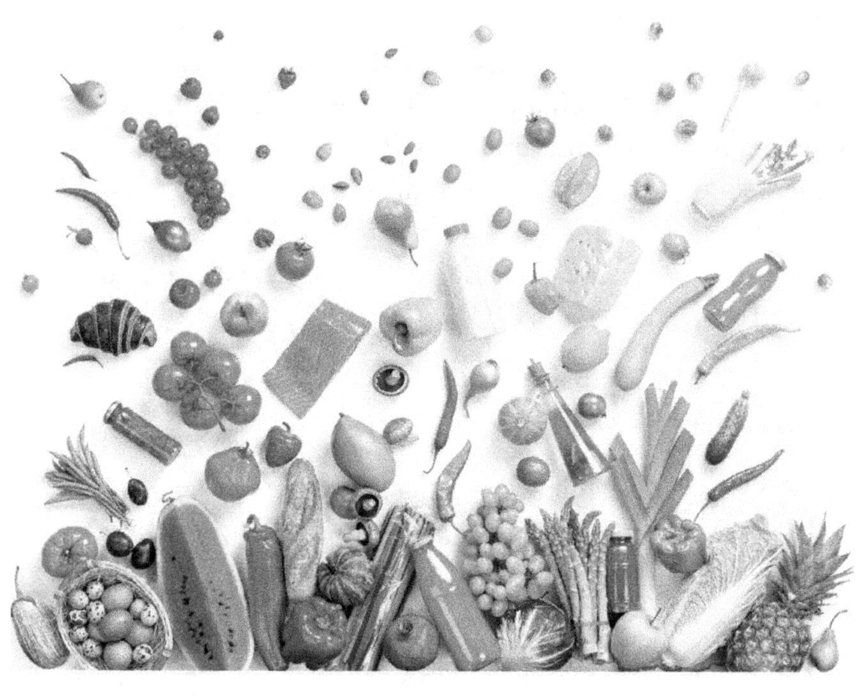

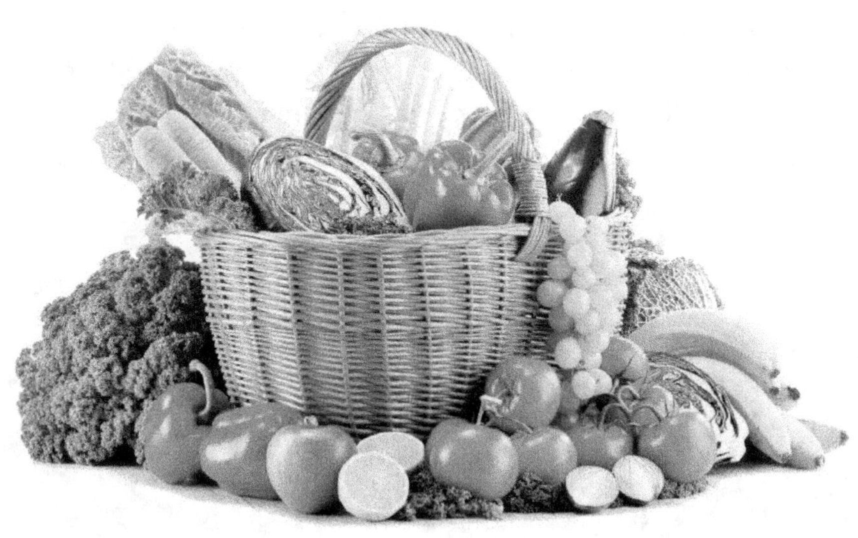

Chapter Five

Breakfast Meal Ideas While Pregnant

These delicious breakfast ideas will help you get your day started right and will encourage you to consume one or two of your daily five servings before leaving the house.

Apple in Oats Brand.

Servings: 2

Ingredients

- 200 mL semi-skimmed milk.
- 50 grams of oatmeal
- 1 dessert apple diced with cinnamon (1 pinch)

Method

- In a saucepan, bring the milk, porridge oats, and dessert apple to a boil.
- Simmer at a lower temperature, stirring frequently.
- Serve the porridge with a pinch of cinnamon on top.

An Oat-Topped Banana Smoothie.

(My favorite Fruit) Servings: 2

Ingredients

- 100 mL semi-skimmed milk
- 2 tablespoons oats

Method

- Peeled, chopped bananas should be added to blenders.

- After adding the milk, add the oats to the blender.
- Blend until the mixture is frothy and smooth before serving.

One Slice of Toast with Mashed Avocado and Tomato.

Servings: 2

Ingredients

- 1 ripe avocado
- 5 sliced cherry tomatoes with lemon juice
- A few basil leaves on any toast you want

Method

- First, remove the avocado stone and place it in a bowl.
- Mash the avocado in the bowl with a fork.
- Add a squeeze of lemon juice to taste.
- After scooping the tomatoes, basil, and avocado onto the toast, combine them.
- For an extra kick, add some balsamic vinegar to the mashed avocado, tomato, and basil.

Berry Smoothie

Servings: 2

Ingredients

- 150 g strawberries, hulled and sliced
- 125g raspberries, 75 mL thick vanilla yogurt in 150 mL
- 4 cubes of ice

Method

- Blend the berries, milk, yogurt, and ice cubes in a blender.
- Blend the mixture until smooth and frothy before serving.

Crunchy Oat and Nut Yogurt

Servings: 6

Ingredients

- Rolled oats 90g olive oil,
- 1 tbsp maple syrup,
- 2 tbsp
- 100g dried fruit of your choice (raisins, apricots, apples)
- 50g chopped pecans 50g chopped almonds (blanched)

Method

- In a mixing bowl, combine the oats, maple syrup, and oil.
- Preheat the oven to 180°C.
- Spread the oat mixture onto a baking sheet and bake for 5 minutes.
- Then, sprinkle the nuts on top of the oat mixture and bake for 5 minutes, stirring once, or until the nuts appear crunchy.
- After transferring to a bowl, add the dried fruit. Choose a yogurt to go on top.

Strawberry and Blueberry Overnight Oats.

Servings: 4

Ingredients

- 50g porridge rolled oats
- 1 cup milk, 2 tablespoons yogurt

- 50g strawberries and blueberries, cut
- Cinnamon pinch

Method

- The oats must be combined with 100ml of milk and cinnamon the night before they are to be consumed.
- The next morning, add a little more milk to help the oats soften.
- Before serving, stir in the yogurt and berries.

Pumpkin-seeded Seeded Vegan Whole-meal Pretzels

Servings: 3

Ingredients

- To make the dough
- 240 mL soya milk 120 mL hot water
- 1 tablespoon sugar 1 tablespoon dried yeast
- 220 g bread flour (strong white)
- 220 g whole grain flour
- 1 teaspoon salt
- 2 liters of water must be boiled
- 4 tablespoons bicarbonate of soda
- 2 tbsp coarse sea salt to finish
- 4 tablespoons pumpkin seeds

Methods

- To make a tepid mixture, combine the hot water and soya milk. Add the sugar and yeast to this mixture and set aside for 5-6 minutes to activate.
- In a large mixing bowl, combine the bread flour, whole meal flour, and salt. Slowly add the yeast mixture while mixing to form a dough.

- Knead the dough for 5-6 minutes, or until it is elastic. Allow the dough to rise in a warm place for 45-60 minutes, or until it has doubled in size.
- Preheat the oven to 200°C/400°F/Gas Mark 6 and set aside. Then divide the dough into ten equal pieces and roll each into a 40-50cm long sausage.
- Form each sausage into a 'U' shape by twisting the ends together, then folding the ends down to the base of the 'U' and pressing down to seal, resulting in the classic pretzel shape. Rep with the remaining ten pieces.
- Bring the water and baking powder to a boil in a large saucepan. Once the water is boiling, add each pretzel and cook for about 30 seconds before removing it from the water.
- Place the pretzels on a baking sheet and top with sea salt and pumpkin seeds. Place in the oven for 18-20 minutes, or until golden.

Each 82g pretzel contains:

- 1.2g Fat
- 0.2g Saturated fat
- 33g Carbs
- 1.7g Sugars
- 3g Fiber
- 6.1g Protein
- 0.01g Salt

Chickpea and Potato Hash

Servings: 2

Ingredients

- 450 g peeled and diced potato
- 2 tablespoons olive oil
- 3 garlic cloves, puréed
- 1 red bell pepper
- 1 diced red onion
- 100 g sliced chestnut mushrooms

- 1 teaspoon onion powder
- 1/2 teaspoon cumin powder
- 1 tablespoon smoked paprika
- 400 g drained chickpeas
- 1 peeled and sliced avocado
- 100 g spinach, fresh
- A handful of chopped fresh parsley and a pinch of dried chili flakes

Method

- Preheat the oven to 200°C/400°F/Gas Mark 6 and set aside. Bring a pot of water to a boil with the potato. Cook for 10-12 minutes before draining.
- Transfer the potatoes to a baking sheet, drizzle with one tablespoon of oil, and bake for 20-25 minutes, or until crisp and golden.
- Then, in a pan over medium heat, add the remaining oil, garlic, red pepper, onion, chestnut mushrooms, onion powder, cumin, and paprika, and sauté for 3-4 minutes.
- Then add the potato and chickpeas to the pan and cook for 3-4 minutes more. Finally, cook the spinach for 2-3 minutes, or until wilted.
- Finish with the sliced avocado, parsley, and chili flakes.

Each 505g serving contains:

- 23g Fat
- 3.1g Saturated Fat
- 71g Carbohydrate
- 12g Sugars
- 20g Fibre
- 17g Protein
- 1g Salt.

Spanish Omelet

Servings: 2

Ingredients

| **For the additions** | **To make the omelet** |

For the additions

- Olive oil (60 mL)
- 2 yellow medium potatoes
- 0.50-pound medium white onion
- 2 Roma tomatoes, small
- 1 tablespoon Mexican oregano

To make the omelet

- Chickpea flour 170 g
- 2 tablespoons nutritional yeast
- 1 teaspoon black salt
- 300 mL bottled water
- Vegan cheese, grated (optional)

Methods

- First, rinse all of the vegetables and peel the potatoes. Then, thinly slice the peeled potatoes and onions (about 18-inch pieces). Cut the tomatoes into 14-inch coins.
- Preheat the olive oil in a medium frying pan over medium-low heat. Stir in the potatoes to coat with the oil. Cook for 10 minutes, stirring frequently to ensure even cooking.
- Then, combine the sliced onions and mix well. Cook for another 5-6 minutes, stirring constantly to prevent the potatoes and onion from browning too much.
- Continue stirring while adding the oregano and cooking for 3-4 minutes more. Then, remove the potato-onion mixture from the heat and strain the oil into a bowl (reserve it to cook the whole omelet in). Set aside the mixture to cool.
- Meanwhile, in the same pan over medium heat, fry your tomato slices. Cook the tomatoes until they are browning on both sides, about 2-3 minutes per side. Set them aside after removing them from the pan.

Omelette

- After you've finished preparing the vegetables, return the frying pan to medium-low heat and add the reserved olive oil.
- In a medium mixing bowl, combine the chickpea flour, nutritional yeast, black salt, and water until no lumps remain. Stir in the potato-onion mixture, and then spoon half of the batter into the frying pan.
- Layer the tomato slices evenly on top, then sprinkle with optional vegan cheese.
- Spread the remaining batter evenly over the tomatoes and cheese. Gently work your way around the omelet with a spatula to push the edges in.
- Cook the omelet for 5-6 minutes, or until the top is no longer wet (tip: cover your frying pan for the first 1-2 minutes to help it cook evenly).
- To flip the omelet, cover the frying pan with a plate that extends slightly beyond the edges. Flip the frying pan over quickly with your hand on the plate to release the omelet.
- Return your frying pan to the heat and carefully place the omelet back into it. Cook for 5 minutes more, or until the omelet is no longer soft in the center.
- Using the same flipping technique as in step 11, remove your omelet from the pan.
- Allow the omelet to rest for about 10-15 minutes before cutting.

Cacao and Hazelnut Spread Vegan

Servings: 2

Ingredients

- Hazelnuts (225 g)

- 4 tablespoons maple syrup

- Tinned coconut milk (120 ml)
- 3 tbsp cacao powder

Methods

- Preheat the oven to 180°C/355°F/Gas 4 and set aside.
- Place the hazelnuts on a baking sheet and toast for 15 minutes, or until they begin to brown.
- Blend the hazelnuts, maple syrup, coconut milk, and cacao in a food processor until smooth, which could take up to 8 minutes. To ensure a smooth spread, scrape down the sides regularly.
- Place in a jar and place in the fridge to thicken.

Pancake Recipe with Vegan Peanut Butter and Jam.

- 2 bananas, medium ripe
- 300 mL dairy-free milk, 280 g self-raising flour
- Nush Natural Almond Yoghurt 100 mL
- 150 g Nush cream cheese, 1 teaspoon vanilla extract
- 80 g peanut butter, smooth
- 55 milliliters of maple syrup
- 300 g raspberries, fresh or frozen
- Toppings: crushed peanuts
- Cooking oil of choice for pancakes.

Methods

- To begin, mash the bananas in a bowl. Combine the flour, milk, yogurt, and vanilla extract.
- Heat a teaspoon of oil of choice in a large nonstick pan over medium heat.

- Add 2 tablespoons of pancake batter to make 1 pancake once the oil is hot. Drop from a great height to help create a round pancake.
- Cook for a few minutes before carefully turning over.
- Repeat with the rest of the batter. Add as many pancakes as your pan can hold. Place the cooked pancakes under a warm grill to keep them warm while you finish the rest of the pancakes.
- Meanwhile, heat the raspberries in a saucepan over medium heat and allow them to stew.
- In a separate bowl, combine the cream cheese, peanut butter, and maple syrup.
- When the pancakes are done, plate them. Spread the peanut butter cream cheese mixture on top, followed by the stewed berries. Sprinkle it with crushed peanuts and serve.

Vegan Fluffy Pancakes with Raspberry Sauce

Servings: 2

Ingredients

- To make the pancakes:
- 250 g unbleached flour
- 1 tablespoon bicarbonate of soda
- 1 teaspoon baking powder
- 1 teaspoon salt
- Oat milk 350 mL
- Cooking lubricant
- To make the raspberry sauce:
- Raspberries 400 g
- 2 tablespoons maple syrup
- 1 tablespoon vanilla extract

Methods

- In a mixing bowl, whisk together the flour, bicarbonate of soda, baking powder, and salt. Then slowly whisk in the oat milk until it forms a thick pancake texture.

- 1 tsp. oil in a pan, and once hot, ladle out the mixture into a pancake.
- Reduce the heat to low and cook for 3-4 minutes, or until bubbles appear. Cook for another 2-3 minutes on the other side.
- Remove from the heat and continue until all of the pancake mix has been used. Throughout the process, you may need to re-oil the pan.
- Meanwhile, blitz the raspberries, maple syrup, and vanilla extract in a food processor until smooth.
- Pour the mixture through a cheesecloth (or fine strainer) into a jug and serve over pancakes.

Vegan Pancakes with Fried 'Egg,' Crispy 'Bacon,' and Spinach

Servings: 2

Ingredients

To make the pancakes:

- 1 cup of flour
- 2 tablespoons organic sugar
- 1 tablespoon baking powder
- 0.50 teaspoon salt
- 1 cup non-dairy milk
- 1 tablespoon of apple cider vinegar
- 1 teaspoon vanilla
- **To make the egg yolk:**
- 0.30 cup peeled and cut sweet potato into small chunks
- 2 tablespoons nutritional yeast
- 1 tablespoon cornstarch
- 1 tablespoon plant-based milk
- 1 tablespoon sunflower oil
- 0.25 cup liquid
- 1 teaspoon Kala Namak (Black Salt) (adds eggy taste)

- 0.50 teaspoon turmeric

To make the egg white:

- 0.25 cup non-dairy milk
- 1/4 cup rice flour
- 0.25 cup yogurt made from plants (preferably with no added sugar)

- 1 teaspoon black salt (Kala Namak)

For the garnish:

- This isn't the Bacon Rashers.
- 1 pound spinach
- A lemon wedges

Methods

Pancakes:

- Combine dry ingredients in a large mixing bowl and wet ingredients in a separate mixing bowl.
- Pour the wet mixture into the dry mixture, whisk until smooth, and set aside for 5 minutes.
- Pour 1/2 cup batter into a nonstick skillet set over medium heat. When the top begins to bubble, flip it until it becomes slightly golden in spots. Repeat with the remaining batter.

'The Eggs'

- Boil peeled sweet potato chunks until completely soft in a pan, drain, mash into a pulp, and stir in the remaining egg yolk ingredients.
- Whisk together all of the egg white ingredients in a mixing bowl.
- Heat 2 tbsp of egg white mixture in a frying pan over medium/high heat for 30 seconds to 1 minute.
- 1 tbsp egg yolk mixture in the center of egg white, cover with lid for 2 minutes.
- Repeat with the remaining mixture.

Toppings and Presentation

- In a frying pan, heat 1 tablespoon of oil and fry THIS IS NOT 2 minutes on each side of bacon rashers.
- In a small saucepan with 2 tablespoons water, wilt the spinach.
- Layer the pancakes, then top with spinach, the egg, THIS IS NOT BACON, and drizzle with lemon.

Vegan Crepes with Zesty Orange

Servings: 2

Ingredients

- 125g unbleached flour
- 2 tablespoons soy flour
- A pinch of turmeric
- 2 tablespoons of sunflower or rapeseed oil
- Two oranges
- Agave syrup (75 ml)
- 1/4 teaspoons salt
- 400ml soya Unsweetened drink
- Half a lemon juice
- With additional oil for frying

Method

- To make a smooth batter, whisk together the flours, turmeric, salt, and Provamel Soya Unsweetened.
- Add the oil and mix well.
- In a hot, lightly oiled frying pan, make thin crepes with the mixture. Warm them in a low oven.
- Before cutting the oranges into chunks, peel, segment, and remove the membrane.
- Bring the agave syrup and lemon juice to a boil in a small saucepan.
- Remove from the heat and stir in the orange chunks.

- To serve, place a crepe on a plate, spoon some orange sauce in the center, and fold the crepe over. Serve hot.

Tip

The batter and orange sauce can be made the night before and reheated before serving.

Cinnamon Blueberry Pancakes

Servings: 2

Ingredients:

- Violife Original Creamy 200 g
- Blueberries (200 g)
- 1 tbsp icing sugar 1 tsp. lemon juice
- 150 g unbleached flour
- 2 tablespoons caster sugar 2 tablespoons baking powder pinch of salt
- 1 tablespoon vanilla extract
- 150 mL almond milk, unsweetened
- 0.50 tablespoon vegetable oil
- 1 teaspoon cinnamon

Method

- Place the berries in a small saucepan with the icing sugar and lemon juice and cook for 5-10 minutes on low heat. Keep warm by covering.
- Combine the four, caster sugar, baking powder, and a pinch of salt in the same mixing bowl.
- Whisk together the vanilla extract, cinnamon, and almond milk.
- Heat 2 tsp. oil in a nonstick frying pan over medium heat.
- Cook the pancakes in batches for 3-4 minutes on each side or until cooked, using a heaping tbsp of batter per batch.

- Serve the pancakes with the compote and creamy Violife

Poached Strawberries on Vegan French Toast

Servings: 1

Ingredients

For the strawberries that have been poached

- 120 mL H2O
- Caster sugar (115 g)
- 1 tsp. ground cinnamon 1/2 teaspoon vanilla extract
- 400 g strawberries, fresh

- 1 tablespoon maple syrup
- 1 teaspoon vanilla extract
- 1 teaspoon ground cinnamon
- 1/4 teaspoons ground nutmeg
- 6–8 slices of bread
- 2 tablespoons coconut oil (for frying)
- Each 143g slice contains:

To make the French toast

- Soy milk (240 mL)
- 50 g of flour

Methods

- Bring the water, sugar, vanilla, and cinnamon to a boil in a small saucepan for the poached strawberries.
- Remove from the heat and add the strawberries, making sure they are completely submerged.
- Allow to cool for a few minutes.
- Whisk together the soya milk, gram flour, maple syrup, vanilla extract, cinnamon, and nutmeg for the French toast.
- Pour this into a shallow tray, then place the bread in the batter for one minute before flipping it over for another minute to absorb the mixture.

- Heat the coconut oil in a frying pan over medium heat, then add the bread and fry for 2-3 minutes on each side, or until golden and the batter is cooked through.
- Serve the poached strawberries on top of the French toast.
- To serve, drizzle with the poaching syrup.

Nutritional Information:

5.1g fat, 3.1g saturated fat, 34g carbohydrate, 20g sugars, 3g fiber, 4.3g protein, 0.25g salt.

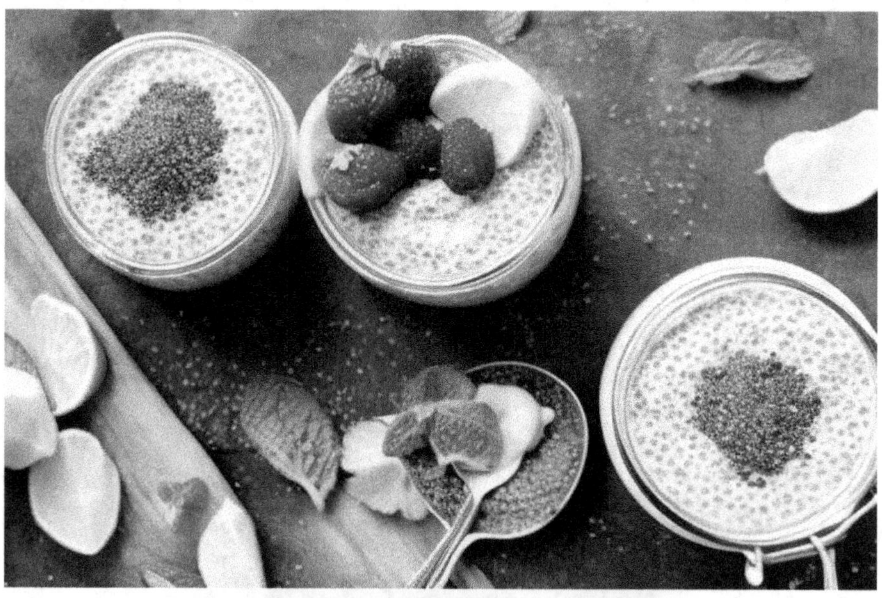

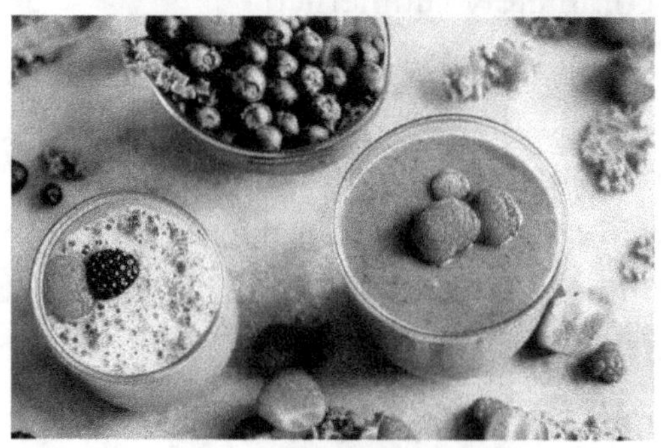

Chapter Six

Lunch Suggestions While Pregnant

Whether you're looking for a quick lunch or a filling dinner, these simple recipes will make meal preparation easier without sacrificing flavor.

Baked Tomatoes on Toast

Servings: 4.

Ingredients

- 8 half-cut tomatoes
- 8 cherry tomatoes, halved
- 2 teaspoons breadcrumbs
- 4 tbsp grated parmesan cheese
- 2 tablespoons chopped fresh chives
- 4 whole meal bread slices

Method

- Begin by preheating the oven to 190°C/Gas 5.
- Place all of the tomatoes on a baking sheet with the cut side up.
- Place the tray in the oven and sprinkle with the chives.
- 10 minutes in the oven.
- Remove the tray from the oven and top with breadcrumbs and parmesan cheese.
- Bake for another 5 minutes, toasting the bread in the meantime.
- Spoon the tomatoes over the toast to serve.

Bacon and Vegetables Frittata

Servings: 2

- 4 beaten medium eggs 2 rashers back bacon, fat removed
- 100g boiled potato (cut into cubes)
- 100g cherry tomatoes, cut in half 125g mushroom, sliced

Method

- Grill the bacon until it is browned on both sides, then flip it over.
- Fry the mushrooms for about 5 minutes over medium heat.
- Cooked bacon should be chopped.
- Fry the potatoes and tomatoes for about five minutes over medium heat.
- In a mixing bowl, combine the eggs, cooked bacon, and mushrooms.
- After that, season and stir in the potatoes and tomatoes.
- Pour the mixture into the frying pan and cook for about 10 minutes on medium heat.
- Place the pan under the grill for two minutes to ensure the frittata is thoroughly cooked.
- To serve, place the frittata on a plate.

Vegan Egg Fried Rice

Servings: 4

Ingredients

- 150g rice
- 2 eggs, whisked 2 bacon rashers, chopped 2 shallots, finely sliced
- 2 tablespoons vegetable oil
- 75g frozen peas

Method

- Bring a saucepan of water to a boil and cook the rice according to the package directions.

- Heat the oil in a wok before adding the whisked eggs.
- Cook until the eggs are set, then remove from the wok and cut into strips.
- Cook the bacon in the wok until it is golden.
- Cook for four minutes after adding the rice, shallots, and peas to the pan.
- Stir in the egg until it is heated through, then serve.

Herb Omelette

Servings: 1

Ingredients

- 3 new eggs
- 1 tbsp. butter
- 1/2 tsp. Extra virgin olive oil
- · Herbs like chives or basil

Method

- Whisk the eggs together and season with salt and pepper to taste.
- In a frying pan, combine the butter and oil.
- Add the whisked eggs once the butter is hot and frothy.
- Move the omelet with a spatula as it cooks to allow any remaining raw egg to cook.
- When the omelet is done, sprinkle with the herbs of your choice and serve.

Vegetable Soup

Servings: 4

Ingredients

- 600ml of milk

- 400ml reduced salt chicken or vegetable stock
- 1 carrot, peeled and diced 1 medium potato, peeled and diced 1 onion, peeled and chopped 1 tablespoon corn flour

Method

- In a large saucepan, combine the stock and vegetables.
- Bring the pan to a boil and continue to cook until the vegetables are tender (approximately 25 minutes).
- Mix the corn flour and 3 tablespoons of the milk until they form a smooth paste.
- Add the corn flour paste and the remaining milk to the saucepan with the vegetables and stock.
- Stir the pan constantly to combine all of the ingredients and allow the soup to thicken.
- Before serving, season with salt and pepper to taste.

Mediterranean Tray Bake

Servings: 4

INGREDIENTS

- 800g fresh potatoes
- 50 grams of pine nuts
- 1 tbsp pesto basilico
- 1 tablespoon of olive oil
- 1 sliced courgette
- 1 sliced aubergine
- 1 red pepper, peeled and chopped
- 1 yellow pepper, seeds and all, chopped

Method

- To begin, preheat the oven to 200°C/400°F/Gas Mark 6.
- In a large oven dish, combine the potatoes, vegetables, and pine nuts.

- Over the potatoes, vegetables, and pine nuts, drizzle the olive oil.
- Bake for 20 minutes with the tray in the oven.
- Remove the tray from the oven and stir in the pesto before returning it to the oven for another 5 minutes before serving.

Savory Rice

Servings: 4

Ingredients

- 150g rice, long grain (easy cook rice)
- 300ml chicken stock, reduced salt
- 1 medium onion, chopped 100g baby sweet corn, sliced 100g peeled and sliced mushrooms 1 teaspoon curry powder
- 1 tsp. vegetable oil

Method

- In a saucepan, heat the vegetable oil and fry the onions for two minutes.
- Cook for another two minutes after adding the mushrooms to the pan.
- Stir in the rice, followed by the stock, curry powder, and sweetcorn.
- Bring the pan to a boil, then reduce the heat to allow it to simmer.
- Continue to simmer for 20 minutes, adding more water to the pan as needed. Cook until the rice is fully cooked, then serve right away.

Plate with Prosciutto, Mozzarella, and Melon

Servings: 2

Ingredients

- 1 cup cantaloupe cubes
- 6 thin prosciutto slices, cut in half
- 10 fresh mozzarella balls, small
- 1/2 cup halved cherry tomatoes
- 6 whole-wheat baguette slices (1/4 inch thick)
- 1/2 cup unsweetened hazelnuts
- 4 strawberries dipped in chocolate (see Tip)

Method

Step 1

- Divide the ingredients evenly between two plates.

Tips

- Want to try your hand at making your chocolate-covered strawberries? Try these decadent Chocolate-Covered Prosecco Strawberries.
- To prepare ahead of time, separate the ingredients into separate table containers.

Nutritional Information

Per Serving: 546 calories; protein 24g; carbohydrates 44g; dietary fiber 6.5g; sugars 16.4g; fat 33.8g; saturated fat 9.7g; cholesterol 52.1mg; vitamin A 3391.4IU; vitamin C 54mg; folate 53.4mcg; calcium 318.1mg; iron 3mg; magnesium 66.2mg; potassium 555.8mg; sodium 936mg; thiamin 0.2mg; added sugar 6g.

Chapter Seven

Vegan Recipe Suggestions for Dinner

Burritos with Vegan Mixed Beans, Chilli, and Rice

Servings: 8

Ingredients

- 1 tablespoon vegetable oil
- 1 onion, finely diced 2 garlic cloves, puréed
- 0.50 teaspoon chili powder
- 1 tablespoon smoked paprika
- 1 teaspoon cumin
- 1 tin 400g mixed beans, drained
- 1 tin chopped tomatoes (400g)
- 240 mL veggie stock
- 175 g rice, cooked according to package directions
- 2 chopped tomatoes 60 g spinach
- 1 peeled and sliced red onion
- 8 flour tortilla wraps

Method

- In a saucepan over medium heat, heat the oil, then add the onion, garlic, dried chili flakes, smoked paprika, and ground cumin and cook for 2-3 minutes.

Cook for 15-20 minutes after adding the beans, chopped tomatoes, and vegetable stock.

- To make the burrito, wrap a tortilla around spinach, rice, beans, tomato, and red onion. To make the burrito, fold the sides in and tightly roll the wrap.

Nutrition facts per serving (183g):

209 calories, 1.9g fat, 0.6g saturated fat, 40.4g carbohydrate, 3.5g sugar, 5.4g fiber, 8.9g protein, 0.68g salt

Cakes with Minty Courgette and Millet

Servings: 3

Ingredients

- 80 grams of millet
- 1 tablespoon bouillon powder
- 1 teaspoon flakes of sea salt
- 240 mL H2O
- 4 green onions
- 1 peeled and grated carrot
- 1 garlic clove, peeled and crushed
- 1 peeled and grated courgette
- 2 tbsp chopped fresh chives
- 2 tbsp freshly chopped mint 3 tbsp gram (chickpea) flour
- To taste, season with sea salt and black pepper.
- To prepare the chia egg
- 3 tablespoons chia seeds in 9 tablespoons water

To fry

- ·A drizzle of vegetable oil

Method

- In a small saucepan, combine the millet, bouillon, salt, and water. Stir once to combine, then bring to a boil. Allow to simmer until all of the water has evaporated and the millet is tender. Place aside to cool.

- Mix in the remaining ingredients, including the chia egg, until thoroughly combined.
- Season with salt and pepper before forming into six equal patties.
- In a shallow frying pan, heat the oil and add the millet cakes. Fry for a few minutes over medium heat, until golden.
- Repeat on the other side until the cakes are piping hot and golden. Serve right away.

Calzone of Vegan Roasted Vegetables with Olives

Servings: 8

Ingredients

To make the dough

- 650 g bread flour (strong white)
- 7 g yeast fact action 3 tsp. salt 2 tbsp olive oil
- 375 mL hot water

To make the filling

- 1 diced courgette
- 155 g black olives, pitted
- 1 large red onion, peeled and cut into wedges
- 1 diced yellow pepper
- 4 garlic cloves, sliced
- 200 g dairy-free cheese, to taste, grated sea salt and black pepper

To make the sauce

- 1 Can (Chopped) Tomatoes
- 2 Teaspoon Sugar
- 1 Tablespoon Dried Italian Herbs
- 4 Crushed Garlic Cloves
- 1 Tablespoon Balsamic Vinegar

- 1 Teaspoon Chilli Flakes
- To Taste, Sea Salt and Black Pepper.

Method

- In a large mixing bowl, combine all of the dry ingredients for the dough. Add the water and oil gradually, mixing with your hands until the mixture forms a soft dough.
- Turn the dough out onto a floured work surface and knead for at least 5 minutes, or until smooth and elastic.
- Return the dough to an oiled bowl, cover with a clean tea towel, and set aside for 1 hour to rise.
- Preheat the oven to 200°C/400°F/Gas Mark 6 and set aside. In a roasting dish, season the vegetables for the filling and drizzle with olive oil. Bake for 30 minutes in a preheated oven.
- In a saucepan, combine all of the sauce ingredients and bring to a gentle simmer. Allow to simmer for 20 minutes, or until slightly reduced.
- Divide the dough into 8 equal portions once it has finished rising. Roll and stretch each ball of dough to a round 9-inch circle on a well-floured surface.
- Spread some tomato sauce, roasted vegetables, and grated cheese on each pizza.
- Fold the dough over the filling crimp and roll the free edges together to completely seal.
- Place the calzones on a flour-dusted baking sheet and bake for 20 minutes, or until golden and puffy.
- Remove from the oven and serve immediately with an additional drizzle of olive oil.

Nutritional info

Fat 2.6g, Saturates 0.4g, Carbohydrates 28g, Sugars 3.0g, Protein 5.0g, Salt 0.23g per 100g serving

Tomato and Pine Nut Salsa with Balsamic Roasted Red Cabbage Steaks

Servings: 4

Ingredients

To prepare the roasted red cabbage

- 1 tablespoon olive oil
- 2 tablespoons agave syrup
- 2 tablespoons balsamic vinegar
- 1 teaspoon garlic salt
- 1 teaspoon dried basil
- 1 head of red cabbage

- 0.50 finely diced red onion
- 1 bunch chopped parsley 3 tbsp olive oil
- 1 tablespoon maple syrup
- 2 tablespoons apple cider vinegar
- 8 cherry tomatoes, quartered 2 tbsp toasted pine nuts

To make the tomato salsa

Method

- Preheat the oven to 180°C/355°F/Gas 4 and set aside. Combine the olive oil, agave, balsamic vinegar, garlic salt, and basil in a mixing bowl.
- Then, cut the cabbage into four 1-inch steaks and coat them in balsamic vinegar with a pastry brush.
- Place them on a baking sheet and roast for 30-40 minutes, or until cooked through.

- Make the tomato salsa while the cabbage roasts. When the cabbage steaks are ready to serve, combine all of the salsa ingredients and spoon over them.

Nutrition facts per serving (298g):

257 calories 14g fat, 2g saturated fat, 31g carbohydrate, 21g sugars, 5g fiber, 3.8g protein, 0.16g salt

Crispy Cauliflower Steak with Homemade Tomato Sauce (Vegan).

Servings: 4

Ingredients

In the case of the steak,

- Soy milk (240 mL)
- 1 tablespoon of apple cider vinegar
- 100 g unbleached flour
- 1 teaspoon garlic powder 65 g corn flour
- 4 tablespoons nutritional yeast
- 1 teaspoon salt
- 1 teaspoon black pepper
- 175 g breadcrumbs (panko)
- 1 cauliflower head, sliced into 4 steaks

To make your tomato sauce

- Plum tomatoes 600 g
- 1 tablespoon oil
- 1 large onion, diced 3 garlic cloves, peeled and chopped
- 2 tablespoons tomato puree
- 1 teaspoon sugar
- 2 tablespoons fresh parsley
- 1 tablespoon fresh thyme, plus salt and pepper to taste

Method

- Preheat the oven to 200°C/400°F/Gas Mark 6 and set aside.
- To make buttermilk, whisk together the soy milk and apple cider vinegar and set aside for 10 minutes.
- Sift the flour and corn flour together in a large mixing bowl, then whisk in the garlic powder, nutritional yeast, salt, and pepper.
- Combine the buttermilk and dry ingredients. To make a wet batter, whisk everything together thoroughly.
- In a separate bowl, combine the panko breadcrumbs.
- Dip each cauliflower steak completely into the wet batter before letting any excess drip off. Then, dip each steak into the panko breadcrumbs, making sure that all sides are evenly coated.
- Cook the steaks in the oven for 40-50 minutes, or until they are cooked through and tender.
- Make the tomato sauce while the steaks are cooking.
- Toss the plum tomatoes in boiling water for 20 minutes, or until the skins begin to peel away.
- Remove the tomatoes' skins, chop them into chunks, and set aside.
- Add the oil to a pan over medium heat and fry the onion for a few minutes until translucent, then add the garlic and fry for a few minutes longer.
- Season with salt and pepper and add the peeled and chopped plum tomatoes, tomato purée, sugar, and herbs.
- Set aside after 20 minutes of simmering.
- Remove the steaks from the oven when they are done.
- Serve with a fresh salad or new potatoes and a heaping spoonful of tomato sauce.

Each 506g serving contains:

6.4g fat, 1g saturated fat, 92g carbohydrate, 11g sugar, 8g fiber, 16g protein, 1.8g salt

Vegan Moroccan Buddha Bowl in the Winter

Servings: 3

Ingredients

- Roasted carrots with cumin
- 1 tablespoon olive oil
- 2 tablespoons maple syrup
- 2 teaspoon cumin seeds
- 3 chopped carrots
- Roasted chickpeas, walnuts, and pumpkin seeds
- 1 tablespoon olive oil
- 1 teaspoon ras el hanout
- 1 can drain chickpeas
- walnuts 60 g
- Pumpkin seeds (30 g)

To make the falafel

- 1 can drain chickpeas
- 1 diced onion
- 1 chopped garlic clove
- 1 teaspoon cumin
- 1 teaspoon coriander powder
- 1 teaspoon ground cinnamon
- 3 tbsp plain flour a handful of chopped parsley
- 180 g Israeli couscous, cooked according to the package
- 1/2 a grated beetroot
- 1 lime, juiced only
- 1 teaspoon cumin
- Yogurt with lime and coriander
- Soya yoghurt (80 mL)
- 1 lime, juiced with only a handful of coriander

To provide

- 150 g kale
- 6 sliced radishes
- 3 tablespoons toasted almond flake

- 3 tablespoons sesame seeds
- 3 spring onions. finely diced

Method

- Preheat the oven to 180°C/355°F/Gas 4 and set aside.
- To make the carrots, combine the oil, maple syrup, cumin seeds, and carrots.
- Place on a baking sheet and bake for 30-35 minutes, or until done. Season with salt and pepper to taste.
- Combine the oil, ras el hanout, chickpeas, and walnuts for the roasted chickpeas, walnuts, and pumpkin seeds.
- Spread out on a baking sheet and bake for 20 minutes.
- Roast for another 10 minutes after adding the pumpkin seeds.
- To make the falafel, combine all of the ingredients in a food processor and blend until a thick paste forms.
- Season with salt and pepper to taste.
- Form into 9 small patties, place on a baking sheet lined with parchment paper, and bake for 15 minutes, or until browned on the outside and cooked through.
- In a mixing bowl, combine all of the ingredients for the beetroot couscous.
- Season with salt and pepper to taste.
- To make the lime and coriander yogurt, whisk together all of the ingredients until smooth, then season to taste.
- To serve, bring a pot of water to a boil, add the kale, and cook for 2-3 minutes before draining.
- In a mixing bowl, layer the carrots, falafel, radishes, chickpea mixture, and couscous.
- Drizzle with yogurt and sprinkle with almonds, sesame seeds, and spring onions.

Squash and Sage Vegan Cheesy Pithivier

Servings: 3

Ingredients

- 0.50 cubed large butternut squash
- 1 large red onion, peeled and cut into wedges
- 12 sage leaves, fresh
- 1 tbsp olive oil plain flour ready-rolled dairy-free puff pastry
- 100 g nondairy cheese
- 60 mL soya milk, unsweetened
- To taste, sea salt and black pepper

Method

- Preheat the oven to 180°C/350°F/Gas Mark 4 and set aside. Arrange the squash, onion, and half of the sage in a baking dish and drizzle with oil to make the pithivier.
- Season to taste, then bake for 30 minutes, or until the squash cubes are tender. Remove from the oven, but leave it on.
- Unroll the pastry sheet and roll it out a little more on a floured surface. Cut out two 23cm diameter circles and place one on a floured baking sheet.
- When the squash has finished cooking and has cooled slightly, taste it and adjust the seasoning as needed. Remove the sage leaves and replace them with fresh, shredded sage. Spoon the squash mixture onto the baking sheet pastry, leaving a 2cm border around the edge.
- Grate the cheese over the squash, avoiding the border. Apply a thin layer of soy milk to the border.
- Place the remaining pastry circle over the filling and seal the edges with a fork.

- Score the top and decorate with pastry shapes cut from the trimmings.
- Place the baking sheet in the oven for 30 minutes, or until crisp and golden.
- Serve hot or cold, wedged with fresh leaves and balsamic glaze.

Nutritional info:

Each 289g serving contains:

40g fat, 13g saturated fat, 7.6g sugars, and 1.2g salt

Stromboli with Vegan Roasted Vegetables

Servings: 8

Ingredients

To make the dough

- 450 g hard white bread
- 1 teaspoon fast-acting yeast
- 4 tablespoons olive oil
- 2 tsp. flakes sea salt
- Hand-hot water, 300 mL

To make the filling

- 1 thinly sliced small aubergine
- 1 thinly sliced courgette
- 2 medium red peppers 2 medium yellow peppers
- 150 g fresh baby spinach
- 6 tbsp red or green dairy-free pesto
- Black olives (75 g)
- 25 g fresh basil leaves, to taste, sea salt and black pepper a little olive oil for brushing

Method

- Preheat the grill to medium, then place the pepper halves on the grill for about 10 minutes, checking them frequently.

- Set the peppers aside to cool enough to peel away the skins once the skins have turned black. Remove and discard the skins before slicing the peppers into thick strips.
- In a large mixing bowl, combine all of the dough ingredients and form a ball with your hands.
- Knead for 5-10 minutes, or until smooth and elastic, on a clean, floured surface.
- Coat the dough lightly with oil and return it to the bowl, loosely covered with a damp tea towel, to rise. This will take about an hour, or until the size has doubled.
- Preheat the oven to 180°C/350°F/Gas Mark 4 and set aside.
- Brush the aubergine and courgette slices with oil and place them on a baking sheet.
- Season with salt and pepper and bake for 15 minutes, or until soft. Keep the oven on.
- Transfer the dough to a floured surface after it has risen and knock out the air.
- Roll out to a large rectangle and spread with pesto, leaving a 5cm border all around. As you go, layer on the cooked vegetables, olives, basil, spinach, and seasoning.
- Fold the two shorter ends of the dough inwards a couple of inches and then roll up to completely encase the filling, beginning with a longer edge.
- Place on a baking sheet, drizzle with olive oil, and season with sea salt.
- Preheat the oven to 400°F and bake for 40 minutes or until golden and puffy.
- Cut into slices and serve hot, warm, or cold.

Nutritional info

For each 100g portion:

Fat (5.3g), Saturates (0.8g), Carbohydrates (22g), Sugars (1.8g), Protein (4.6g), Salt (2.7g).

Risotto with Mushrooms, Leek, and Asparagus

Servings: 4

Ingredients

To make the risotto

- 2 tablespoons dairy-free butter
- 2 tablespoons olive oil
- 1 leek, sliced 2 large shallots, minced 2 garlic cloves, minced 300 g mixed mushrooms, minced 100 g asparagus, sliced
- 2 tablespoons nutritional yeast
- 1.50 liters vegetable broth
- 3 tbsp chopped fresh parsley or chives 300 g arborio rice sea salt and black pepper to taste
- 75 g wild mushrooms, halved 2 tbsp freshly chopped parsley or chives 2 tbsp dairy-free butter
- 1 garlic clove, crushed asparagus tips, sea salt, and black pepper to taste

Method

- Melt the butter and oil in a large, wide frying pan or flameproof casserole dish over medium heat.
- Season the shallots, leeks, garlic, asparagus, and mushrooms and sauté until softened and fragrant.
- Stir everything together in the pan to coat the grains with oil.
- Add a couple of ladles of hot stock to the rice and stir until absorbed.

- Continue adding the stock and stirring until absorbed until the rice is just cooked and the risotto looks starchy and creamy.
- To taste, add the nutritional yeast, herbs, and seasoning.
- In a frying pan, combine all of the serving ingredients and stir fry over high heat until the asparagus is tender and the mushrooms are golden around the edges.
- Top the risotto with the garlic mushroom mixture and drizzle with extra virgin olive oil. If desired, top with nondairy parmesan-style cheese.

Each 100g serving contains:

Carbohydrates 0.8g Saturated Fat 4.7g 22 g of sugars and 1.1g of protein 0.55g salt 4.1g

Vegan Blue Cheese and Broccoli Quiche

Servings: 4

Ingredients

The pastry method

- 150 g dairy-free butter 300 g plain flour
- 1 teaspoon sea salt 2 tablespoons fresh water
- To make the filling
- Vegan blue cheese 100 g
- 100 g broccoli tender stem
- 1 chopped white onion
- 1 tablespoon of dairy-free butter
- Silken tofu 600 g

- 90 g of flour
- 30 g dietary yeast
- 2 tablespoons Dijon mustard
- 2 tbsp fresh parsley, to taste, chopped sea salt and black pepper
- A 25 cm quiche tin,
- A 35cm circle of greaseproof paper,

- Ceramic baking beans, or dried chickpeas/lentils/beans are also required.

Method

- To make the pastry, combine the flour, salt, and butter in a large mixing bowl. Working quickly, lightly rub the butter into the flour with your fingertips until everything is incorporated and the mixture resembles fine breadcrumbs.
- Drizzle in the water and mix with a knife until a dough forms.
- Roll everything into a ball with your hands and wrap it in Clingfilm. Refrigerate the dough for 30 minutes. At this point, the pastry can be frozen for later use.
- While the dough is resting, prepare the filling by blending the tofu, mustard, nutritional yeast, and gram flour with some seasoning in a blender. Process until completely smooth.
- In a frying pan, melt the butter and add the onion.
- Set aside to cool slightly after sautéing the onion until it is soft and translucent.
- Preheat the oven to 170°C/340°F/Gas Mark 3 and set aside.
- Roll out the pastry to a large circle, approximately 35cm in diameter, on a well-floured, flat surface or board.
- Lift the pastry up and onto the quiche tin using the rolling pin. Gently press the pastry into the tin, making sure there is no air trapped underneath.
- Using a sharp knife, trim the pastry to fit the tin and prick the base all over to prevent it from rising in the oven.
- Spread the dried beans or peas over the greaseproof paper and top with the pastry.
- Bake for 20 minutes with the tin in the oven. Once cooked, remove from the oven, discard the paper and beans, and leave the oven on.

- Pour the silken tofu mixture into the pastry case and evenly distribute the cooked onion and blue cheese cubes.
- Sprinkle with parsley and arrange the broccoli spears on top, pushing them into the filling but leaving them visible.
- Place the quiche in the oven and bake for 30-40 minutes, or until the center is just set.
- Allow for a 5-minute cooling period.
- Serve with steamed new potatoes and a crisp salad, hot, warm, or cold. This is also a great addition to any buffet or party table.

Each 100g serving contains:

Carbohydrates 21g, Sugars 1.1g, Protein 10g, Salt 0.75g.

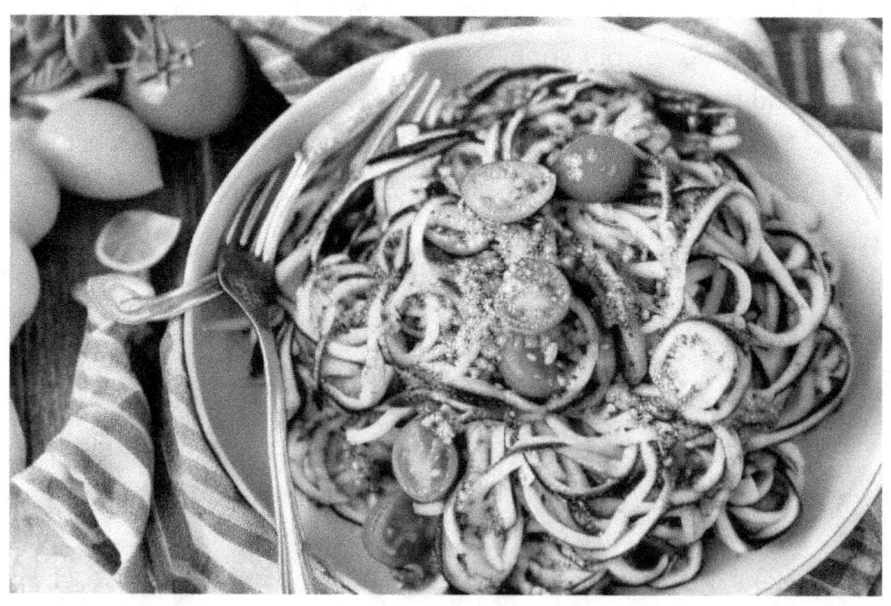

Chapter Eight

Common Complications with Pregnancy

When you are pregnant, your body changes and is influenced by hormones. The changes are required for the baby in your womb to grow and develop. However, changing hormone balances can be problematic and affect expectant mothers in a variety of ways.

Some women report no changes at all, while others report intermittent complaints. Some women experience complaints throughout their pregnancy. The following is a list of the most common symptoms that most pregnant women experience at some point during their pregnancy.

Nausea

Nausea, also known as morning sickness, is a common complaint. It usually begins after the fourth week, when the pregnancy hormones begin to rise. Nausea is most common between weeks seven and ten and then subsides between weeks twelve and fourteen. Some women experience mild nausea, particularly in the morning, while others suffer greatly and may vomit several times per day for some time.

Some women experience severe morning sickness or hyperemesis gravidarum, which causes them to vomit and feel ill throughout their pregnancy. If you have severe morning sickness and persistent vomiting, you may be admitted to the hospital for IV fluids. If you are experiencing severe symptoms, consult with your doctor.

It may reassure you to know that the body always ensures that the baby receives the nutrition it requires to develop. You don't have to be concerned about the baby if you vomit.

While there are no guaranteed cures for nausea, many home remedies are worth a try because they have helped many women manage their symptoms. Here are some pointers:

· If your nausea is worse in the morning, eating something before getting out of bed may help.

· Consume small amounts of food regularly.

· Strong odors should be avoided as they can aggravate nausea.

· Acupuncture is an alternative medicine technique that works for some people.

· If you vomit, it is critical that you drink plenty of fluids to avoid dehydration. Take it easy and try not to be stressed. Before taking any morning sickness medication, always consult your doctor.

Fatigue

Many expectant mothers experience fatigue that is unrelated to a lack of sleep. It is frequently worse at the start of a pregnancy when hormonal changes are most noticeable. You may need to plan a few breaks throughout the day to get through the day and work.

Fatigue combined with nausea can be extremely distressing for some women. It might help to know that the worst of the fatigue is usually followed by a more energetic period in the second trimester. Tiredness is caused by the extra weight of the womb near the end of the pregnancy, and you may have difficulty sleeping. Finding a comfortable sleeping position can be difficult as your belly grows.

Tiredness can also be caused by iron deficiency (anemia). If you want to take iron supplements, talk to your doctor.

Constipation

Constipation and digestive issues are common pregnancy complaints. Because of the pregnancy hormone progesterone, the colon expands and works more slowly. Taking iron supplements while pregnant may also result in constipation. Eating a high-fiber diet rich in vegetables and whole grains can help, but remember to drink plenty of water as well. Walking, water aerobics, yoga, or dance can also help your digestive tract work more efficiently.

Heartburn

Many pregnant women experience acid reflux and heartburn. This is because during pregnancy, muscles that we cannot consciously control relax slightly. One such muscle is the valve that separates the esophagus from the stomach and prevents gastric acid from entering the throat. Avoid extremely fatty, spicy, or smoked foods to prevent or relieve heartburn. You can also try cutting back on coffee and eating smaller meals more frequently. After eating, avoid lying down or bending over straight.

There are also over-the-counter medications that may be beneficial. Consult your doctor about which antacids are appropriate for expectant mothers.

Backache

As your uterus grows heavier, the strain on your muscles, joints, and ligaments increases, particularly in the back and pelvic area. Many pregnant women arch their backs more as their belly grows, putting additional strain on the lower back muscles. It may manifest as a backache that worsens in the latter stages of your pregnancy.

If you have back pain, taking short breaks may help you feel more comfortable and get through the day. Lying on your side with your legs bent and a pillow between your legs and feet is usually relaxing. Because strong muscles are better able to withstand increased strain, the right type of exercise can help prevent back pain.

Urinary tract problems

Feeling the need to urinate and needing to use the restroom more frequently is not always indicative of a problem. During pregnancy, your urine production increases, and the expanding womb puts pressure on your bladder.

When you're pregnant, your chances of getting a urinary tract infection are slightly higher than usual. An infection, if left untreated, can cause premature contractions and, in the worst-case scenario, preterm labor. As a result, it is critical to seek appropriate treatment for any infections. If you need to pee more frequently or if you have burning or pain in your lower belly, see your doctor.

Dental issues

The mucous membranes in your mouth swell and your saliva changes during pregnancy. Your resistance to bacteria decreases as well, which can lead to gum inflammation and cavities. Increased sugar cravings and frequent eating (which often helps with nausea) increase your risk of tooth decay even more. As a result, you should be extra cautious about your oral hygiene while pregnant. Use fluoride toothpaste, rinse with fluoride mouthwash, and floss regularly. When you brush your teeth during pregnancy, your gums may bleed easily. If this occurs, brush more gently.

Congestion in the nose

The amount of blood in the body increases during pregnancy, causing the mucous membranes to swell, thicken, and even bleed more easily. Your nose, mouth, and vaginal mucous membranes are all affected.

For example, you could have a stuffy nose or nosebleeds. Use a saline nasal spray if your nose is congested. This is preferable to over-the-counter nose drops, which can aggravate the problem if used for more than a week. Many pregnant women experiences discomfort for several months, which is why saline is preferable (the other drops are good for a shorter cold, for example).

When you lie down, the swelling in your nose often worsens, and it is common to snore more during pregnancy. If you have snoring issues, try elevating your head with a couple of extra pillows.

Legs and feet swollen

Because you carry more fluid when pregnant, your legs, feet, and hands may swell easily. Any extra fluid collects at your arms and legs' extremities. It can be difficult to put on shoes or wear rings as your belly grows larger. The symptoms are frequently exacerbated after a long day at work or during the summer months when the weather is warm. Wearing compression stockings or sleeping with your legs raised reduces swelling. If you wear compression stockings, put them on first thing in the morning, before the fluid in your legs has accumulated

Discharge from the cervix

Excessive vaginal discharge is common during pregnancy and is caused by increased blood flow to the tissues inside your vagina, which allows fluid to discharge more easily. The discharge is usually milky white and has no odor. Itching, burning, or a strong odor, on the other hand, may indicate an infection.

Contact your doctor if you experience any of these symptoms.

Having difficulty sleeping

Nighttime sleep is frequently disrupted as your belly grows, and many women wake up frequently, leaving them tired. More trips to the bathroom are common, and back and pelvic pain may cause you to change your sleeping position frequently. Sleeping on your side is typically the most comfortable position. Make use of plenty of pillows and keep your bedroom cool. If your nighttime sleep is severely disrupted, try taking short naps to compensate for lost sleep.

Bleeding in the cervix

Early pregnancy vaginal bleeding can be concerning, but light bleeding does not always indicate a problem.

Swollen mucous membranes, mild uterine bleeding, the placenta lying low in the uterus (known as low-lying placenta or placenta previa), vaginal infections, or miscarriage are all possible causes of pregnancy bleeding. Most miscarriages happen before week 12, and some women don't even realize they're pregnant because they mistake the bleeding for a regular period.

However, if you experience pain while bleeding or if there is a large amount of blood, you should always contact your healthcare provider. If you experience vaginal bleeding during the second trimester, seek medical attention right away.

Varicose veins

Pregnancy puts additional strain on your veins, which are the vessels that carry blood back to your heart. During pregnancy, the muscular walls of your blood vessels relax, causing blood to pool and the vessels to swell, while the pressure on veins increases. A varicose vein is an unusually swollen vein. Varicose veins are most commonly found on the legs and calves, but they can also be found around the vagina.

Compression stockings may alleviate symptoms by improving blood circulation in the body. You can also reduce swelling and make your legs feel lighter by raising your legs on a chair or a couch pillow regularly. Some varicose veins disappear completely after pregnancy.

Hemorrhoids

Hemorrhoids are a common complaint that can be inconvenient but are usually not harmful. Hemorrhoids can cause bleeding, burning, or itching around the anus.

Constipation during pregnancy frequently worsens the symptoms. After using the restroom, wash your bottom with water and gently pat the area dry. Medicine is available to relieve pain and itching in severe cases but always consult your health care provider first.

Dizziness

Dizziness is common, especially at the start of a pregnancy when blood pressure is often low. This is due in part to diluted blood and in part to the hormone progesterone relaxing the vascular walls.

If your blood pressure is extremely low, you may feel dizzy, especially if you stand up quickly or after sitting for an extended period. A severe iron deficiency can also cause dizziness. If you take iron supplements, your symptoms may improve.

When you lie on your back, you may feel dizzy, as if you are about to faint, because the heavy uterus weighs down and presses on a large blood vessel called the vena cava. This is referred to as vena cava syndrome. This can be avoided by not lying flat on your back.

Pre-eclampsia

Your blood pressure will rise again during the second half of your pregnancy. If it becomes too high, it may indicate pre-eclampsia. Although this is not a common pregnancy complaint, it is critical to recognize the symptoms. You may experience some of the following symptoms if you have preeclampsia:

- Headache
- Vision shifts
- Ache beneath your right rib cage
- Vomiting and nausea
- Feeling generally ill due to sudden swelling of your hands, feet, or face

Pre-eclampsia is a condition in which you become hypersensitive to particles from the child and the placenta. Typically, the condition is discovered during a routine blood test. Most women with pre-eclampsia have a mild form that can be treated, but some may require hospitalization for emergency care. If you have one or more of the symptoms listed above, contact your doctor.

Skin modifications

Pregnancy hormones affect the skin's elastic tissue, causing pink, red, or purplish streaks to appear as the skin stretches. Stretch marks are commonly found on the belly, breasts, and thighs. Stretch marks fade after birth and turn silvery-gray, but they rarely disappear entirely. During pregnancy, your skin may become more pigmented, resulting in brown patches on your face and body. When you expose your skin to the sun, you increase your chances of developing brown patches, so be cautious and take precautions.

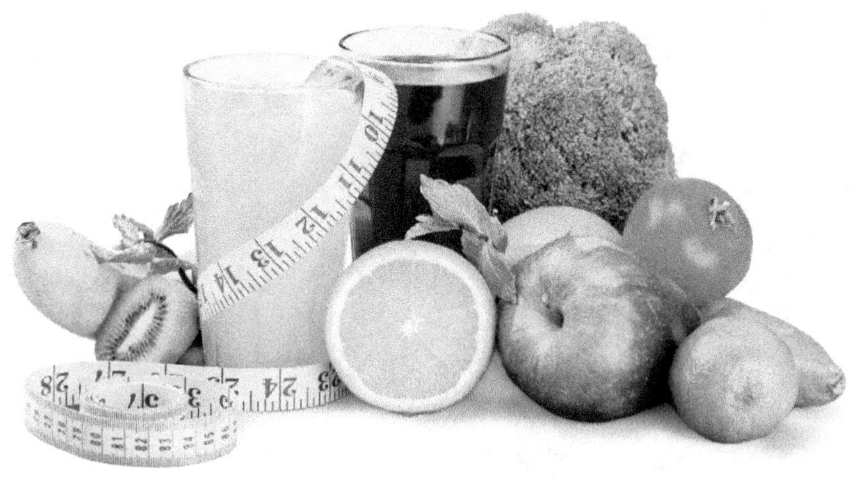

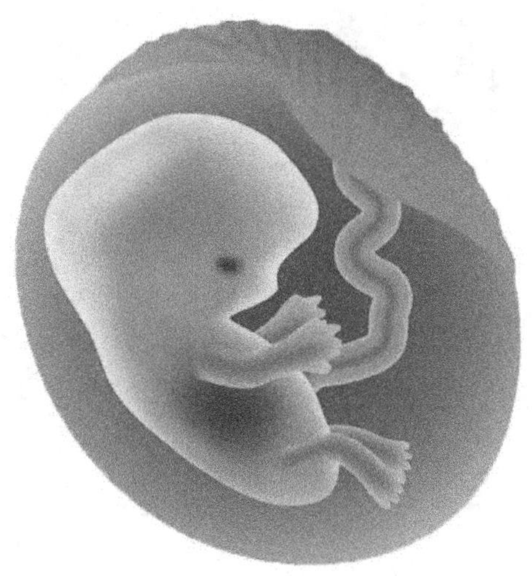

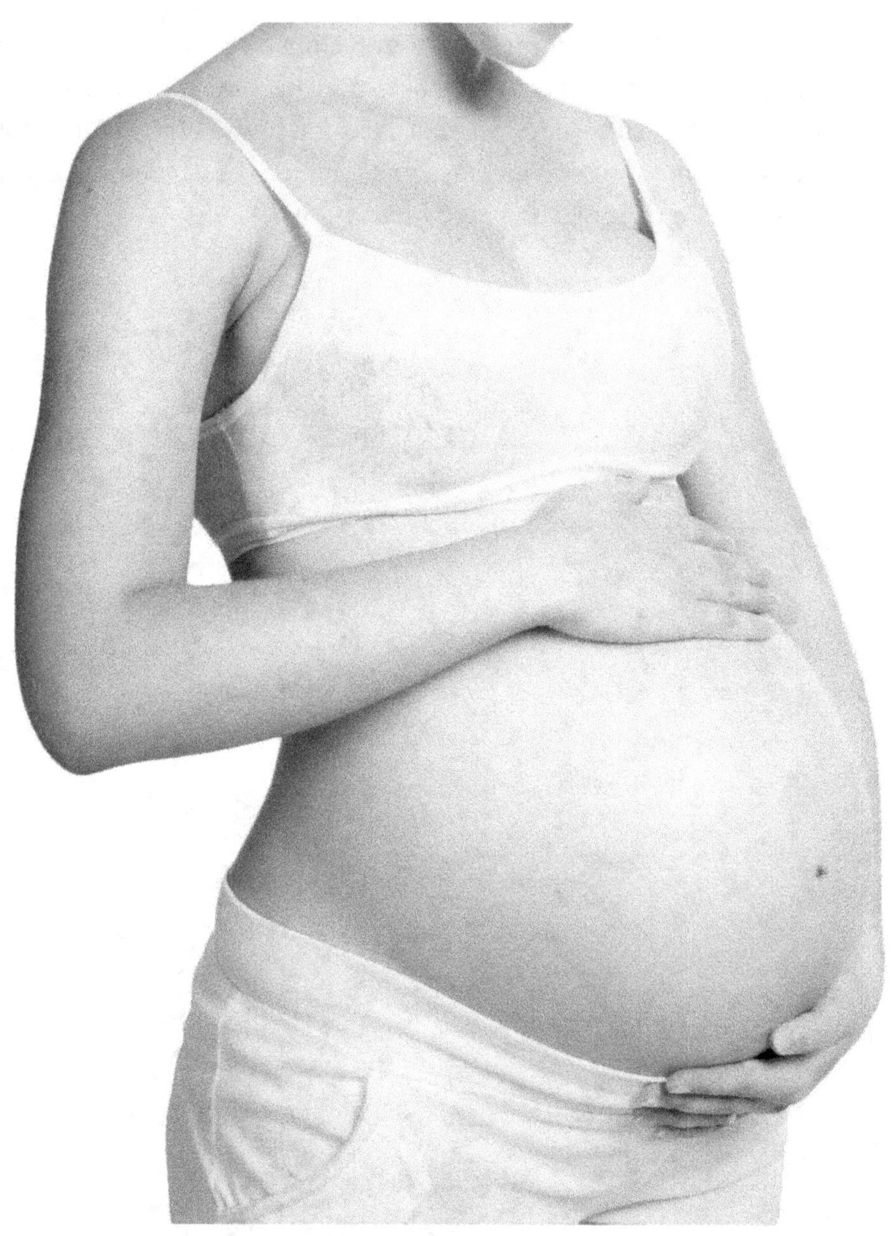

Chapter Nine

Exercises In Relationship with Pregnancy

Exercises for cardio and strength conditioning should be advocated for all pregnant women who are experiencing no difficulties as part of a healthy lifestyle. Maintaining a healthy level of fitness during pregnancy without attempting to reach peak fitness should be an aim of aerobic conditioning in pregnancy.

Understand what:

- The advantages of exercising when pregnant
- Exercise and the pregnancy-related alterations
- Recommendations for exercise during pregnancy
- Activities for fitness recommended during pregnancy
- Exercise precautions during pregnancy
- Pregnancy exercises to stay away from
- Exercises for the pelvic floor and pregnancy
- Workout for the abdomen during pregnancy
- Warning symptoms of pregnancy and exercise
- How to receive assistance.

Women who exercise while pregnant may experience a variety of health advantages, such as better weight management, happier moods, and maintaining fitness levels. Pregnancy-related problems including pre-eclampsia and pregnancy-induced hypertension can be reduced by regular exercise during pregnancy. Consult your doctor, physiotherapist, or other healthcare provider before working out while pregnant.

If you didn't exercise much before becoming pregnant, you may need to adapt your current exercise regimen or pick a new one that suits your needs.

Advantages Of Exercising When Pregnant

Pregnancy exercise has numerous psychological and physical advantages. While managing some pregnancy symptoms, exercise can also help you feel better because it benefits both you and your unborn child.

Regular activity throughout your pregnancy has several advantages, such as:

- Enjoyment
- Enhanced vigor
- Enhanced fitness
- Lower risk of pregnancy issues such as pre-eclampsia and pregnancy-induced hypertension preparedness for the physical demands of labor lower risk of complications during delivery quicker post-labor recovery
- Urinary incontinence prevention and treatment
- Better posture better circulation
- Weight management
- Stress reduction
- Decreasing the danger of anxiety and depression

The ability to handle the physical demands of parenthood was increased by better sleep and the management of insomnia.

Exercise and pregnancy-related alterations

While you are pregnant, your body will alter significantly.

Some of them will hinder your capacity to exercise or force you to change your exercise regimen, such as:

- Relaxing and other hormones loosen ligaments, which could raise your risk of suffering a joint injury (such as sprains).
- You will gain weight as the pregnancy goes along, and your body shape and weight distribution will alter.
- The body's center of gravity shifts as a result, which might affect your balance and coordination.
- Don't calculate the intensity of your workout using your target heart rate because being pregnant causes an increase in your resting heart rate.
- Exercise intensity can be measured in healthy pregnant women using a technique called the Borg's Rating of Perceived Exertion (RPE) scale. This gauges how difficult you feel your body is working.

To prevent dizziness during the second trimester, it is crucial to avoid abrupt changes in position, such as going from reclining to standing and back again.

Recommendations for Exercise During Pregnancy

Pre-exercise screening is used to identify individuals who may be more likely to experience a health issue when engaging in physical activity due to their underlying medical issues.

It serves as a filter or "safety net" to assist in determining if your hazards and benefits from exercise outweigh each other. Before starting a new physical activity or exercise program, go through the pre-exercise self-screening tool.

If you were physically active before becoming pregnant and have been given the all-clear to exercise, it is advised that you:

- On most days of the week, if not all of them, engage in moderate-intensity physical exercise for at least 30 minutes.
- Use your body as a map. When you can talk regularly (but cannot sing), you are exercising at a good intensity, and you don't tire out too rapidly.
- Maintain this level of exercise throughout your pregnancy, or until it becomes difficult for you to do so if you are healthy and are not having any pregnancy issues.
- Observe the recommendations of your doctor, physiotherapist, or other healthcare professional.
- If you were inactive before becoming pregnant but have been given the all-clear to exercise:
- Build up to moderate-intensity exercise by beginning with low-intensity exercises like walking or swimming.
- On most days of the week, if not all of them, try to engage in moderate-intensity physical exercise for at least 30 minutes.
- Start with separate sessions that are each 15 minutes long and work your way up to lengthier sessions.
- Use your body as a map. When you can talk regularly (but cannot sing), you are exercising at a good intensity, and you don't tire out too rapidly.
- Maintain this level of exercise throughout your pregnancy, or until it becomes difficult for you to do so if you are healthy and are not having any pregnancy issues.
- Follow the advice of your physician, physiotherapist, or other healthcare specialist.

Activities for Fitness Recommended During Pregnancy

Even for beginners, the following are generally risk-free activities to engage in while pregnant:

- Cycling while outside or on a stationary bike, walking, swimming
- Exercises that improve the muscles used in jogging, such as pelvic floor exercises
- Workout in the water (aquarobics)
- Stretching, yoga, and other floor workouts
- Pregnancy Pilates workout classes.

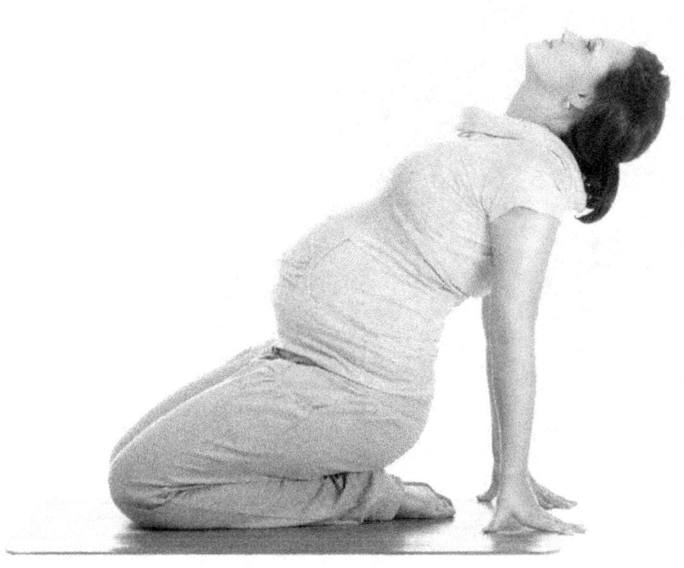

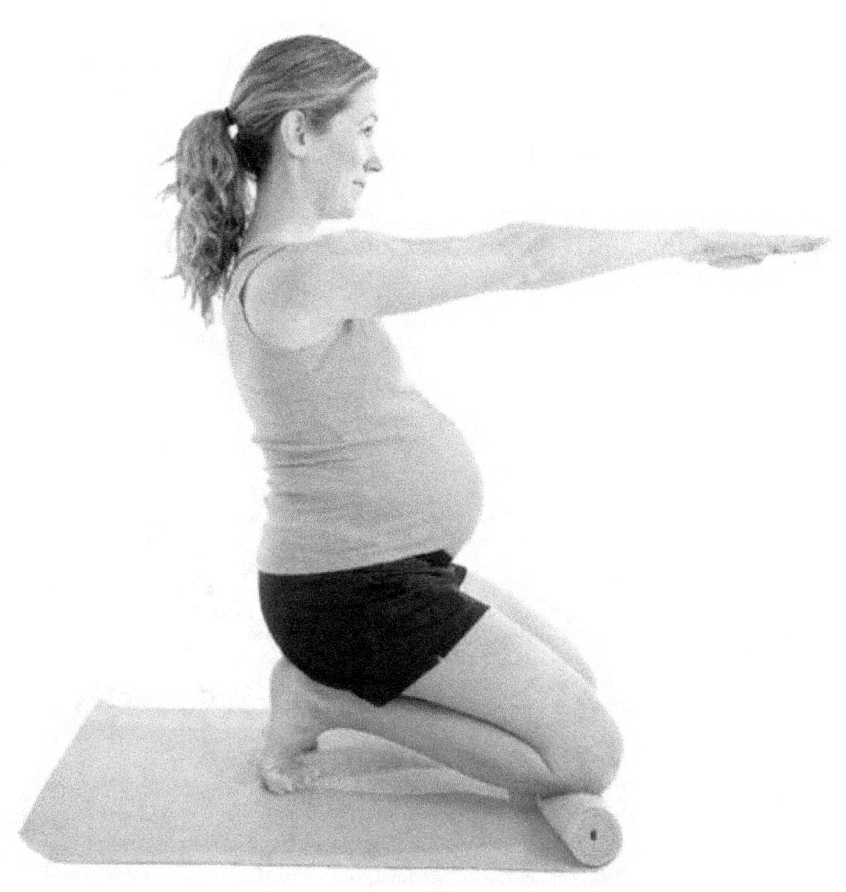

Conclusion

Exercise precautions during pregnancy

While the majority of workouts are risk-free, some of them entail positions and motions that could be dangerous or uncomfortable for expectant mothers.

Follow the advice of your doctor or physiotherapist, but note the following general cautions:

- Avoid overheating your body by, for example, working out until you start to perspire heavily or soaking in hot pools. Reduce the intensity of your activity on hot, sticky days.
- Don't overwork yourself throughout your workout; keep yourself hydrated.
- When weight training, choose for moderate weights and medium to high repetitions; avoid using heavy weights at all costs.
- When stretching, be mindful not to overdo it.
- Exercise should be avoided if you are sick or have a fever.
- If you don't feel like working out on any particular day, don't! It's essential to pay attention to your body to avoid unnecessarily using up your energy.
- When you are pregnant, don't up the ante on your exercise regimen, and always keep your heart rate under 75% of the maximum.

- Additionally, consult your doctor or midwife before continuing or restarting your fitness routine if you get sick or experience a pregnancy issue.

Pregnancy Exercises to Stay Away From

Avoid sports and activities that carry a higher risk of, or are characterized by:

- Extreme balance, coordination, and agility—like in gymnastics—abdominal trauma or pressure, such as from weightlifting, contact or collision, such as from martial arts, soccer, basketball, or other competitive sports, and hard projectile objects or striking implements, like from hockey, cricket, or softball.
- The weight of the baby can hinder the return of blood to the heart during supine workouts (laying on your back), heavy lifting, high-altitude training, and other substantial pressure changes; some of these exercises can be reduced by lying on your side and performing wide squats or lunges.
- Consult your healthcare provider if you're unsure whether a certain activity is safe during pregnancy.

Exercises for the Pelvic Floor and Pregnancy

Since pregnancy and childbirth (by vaginal delivery) weaken your pelvic floor muscles, it is crucial to start exercising them as soon as you learn what you are expecting.

A physiotherapist may recommend the right workouts. These should be continued throughout your pregnancy and resumed as soon as it is convenient after giving birth.

Workout for the Abdomen During Pregnancy

Your spine is supported by sturdy abs. The abdominal muscles of the pelvic floor and internal core function as a built-in "corset" to support the pelvis and lumbar spine.

Women frequently experience diastasis recti abdominis, or abdominal separation, during pregnancy. This condition is characterized by a painless splitting of the abdominal muscle at the midline. Traditional crunches or sit-ups may make this issue worse and are ineffective while pregnant.

To develop the abdominal muscles during pregnancy, appropriate core stability activities are advised. For instance:

- Draw your belly button toward your spine with all of your attention.
- Draw your belly in while exhaling.
- Hold the posture while counting to ten. Breathe deeply and unwind.
- As frequently as you can throughout the day, repeat 10 times.
- This exercise can be done while seated, standing, or on your hands and knees.

Warning Symptoms of Pregnancy and Exercise

Stop exercising right away and visit a doctor if you encounter any of the following during or after physical activity:

- Headache, faintness, or dizziness, heart palpitations
- A chest aches
- Face, hands, or foot swelling
- Contractions with vaginal bleeding and calf ache
- Profound pelvic, pubic, or back discomfort
- Lower-abdominal cramps difficulty walking
- A strange shift in your infant's motion
- Leaking of amniotic fluid, extraordinary breathlessness, extreme exhaustion, and muscle weakness.